MW01484567

Man
Cancer
SEX

By Anne Katz, RN, PhD

Hygeia Media
An imprint of the Oncology Nursing Society
Pittsburgh, Pennsylvania

ONS Publishing Division
Publisher: Leonard Mafrica, MBA, CAE
Director, Commercial Publishing: Barbara Sigler, RN, MNEd
Managing Editor: Lisa M. George, BA
Staff Editor: Amy Nicoletti, BA
Copy Editor: Laura Pinchot, BA
Graphic Designer: Dany Sjoen

Man Cancer Sex

Library of Congress Control Number: 2009934576

ISBN: 978-1-890504-87-8

Publisher's Note
This book is published by Hygeia Media, an imprint of the Oncology Nursing Society (ONS). ONS neither represents nor guarantees that the practices described herein will, if followed, ensure safe and effective patient care. The recommendations contained in this book reflect ONS's judgment regarding the state of general knowledge and practice in the field as of the date of publication. The recommendations may not be appropriate for use in all circumstances. Those who use this book should make their own determinations regarding specific safe and appropriate patient-care practices, taking into account the personnel, equipment, and practices available at the hospital or other facility at which they are located. The editors and publisher cannot be held responsible for any liability incurred as a consequence from the use or application of any of the contents of this book. Figures and tables are used as examples only. They are not meant to be all-inclusive, nor do they represent endorsement of any particular institution by ONS. Mention of specific products and opinions related to those products do not indicate or imply endorsement by ONS. Web sites mentioned are provided for information only; the hosts are responsible for their own content and availability. Unless otherwise indicated, dollar amounts reflect U.S. dollars.

ONS publications are originally published in English. Publishers wishing to translate ONS publications must contact the ONS Publishing Division about licensing arrangements. ONS publications cannot be translated without obtaining written permission from ONS. (Individual tables and figures that are reprinted or adapted require additional permission from the original source.) Because translations from English may not always be accurate or precise, ONS disclaims any responsibility for inaccuracies in words or meaning that may occur as a result of the translation. Readers relying on precise information should check the original English version.

Printed in the United States of America

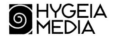

An imprint of the Oncology Nursing Society

For Alan,
a most honorable, ethical, and compassionate man,

and for Zak,
who one day will be all that
and more

Contents

Preface

Over the years, I have worked with many men. Some have been my patients, and I have been honored by the trust they placed in me. Others have been my colleagues, and of these, some have become friends. I have always been fascinated by what makes them male and how they portray themselves in words and deeds. I often joke that I would like to be a man, just for three days, and I would not shave the entire time! But underneath the joke is some truth. It would be fascinating to be a man, just for a while.

I am not sure that men and women really do come from different planets, as the popular media will have us believe. I think we just see life through a slightly different lens that has been honed by personal experience, societal expectations, and a whiff of hormones. We live with and among each other, and I am excited by the dance we perform as we circle each other each and every day.

This book is written for men and for the women and men who love them and live with them through the cancer experience and beyond. For the past five years, I have spent a great deal of my work life trying to understand the hundreds of men who have been patients of mine at CancerCare Manitoba. Just when I think I understand, one of them surprises me. Perhaps it is his use of humor about something that to an outsider would not be that funny. I am allowed to observe how he sees the humor in the situation, and I am grateful for that permission. Or maybe a man allows me to see how deeply devastated he is by his cancer, and I am humbled by his personal tragedy. I have learned about my own humanity through them all.

PART ONE

Understanding the Basics

Why is sex important for us as individuals and as couples? How do we become sexual beings, and what influences this? These introductory chapters will set the stage for the rest of the book by describing the anatomy of the sex organs as well as how things work.

CHAPTER 1

Why Sex Matters

Why is sex important for us as individuals and as couples? How do we become sexual beings, and what influences this? This introductory chapter will set the stage for the rest of the book by defining sex and sexuality in the context of human development across the life span.

Sex, sex, sex—we hear so much about this every day and in every way. Sex sells cars and vacations and clothing. Many men think that they are not having enough sex and that everyone is having more sex than them. We learn how to be sexual from many different sources: parents, peers, school, religious institutions, and the media. What we learn as we grow from childhood into old age (and this learning should and does continue along the life span) may affirm that sex is a good and pleasurable thing if we are lucky or may be less positive if we are not.

The media tend to portray men as testosterone-driven, unfeeling and uncommunicative, stupid and bumbling characters similar to Homer Simpson. Men are portrayed as sexual machines, ready and able to have sex no matter what the circumstances (even with bombs falling around one's ears) or the situation. Many men have integrated these images and are worried when they seem to fall short of them. When illness happens, particularly a life-threatening illness such as cancer, many men don't know what will happen to them sexually.

Sexuality Across the Life Span

Adolescence

As you will learn in the following chapter, sexual development is under the influence of hormones, mostly testosterone for boys. During adolescence, a period of physical growth and development, the boy/young man begins to experience changes to his body that eventually lead to the typical size, shape, and structures of the adult male. The penis and testicles enlarge, hair grows seemingly all over, and the voice deepens. The shoulders grow broader and the hips narrow, leading to the typical inverted triangle shape seen in adult men. The young man grows in height and by the end of adolescence is usually the height he will be as an adult.

Emotional maturation happens during this time, too. The peer group becomes more important in the life of the young man. Many young men are physically mature but lack the emotional and social maturity of adults. Their thinking may still be quite immature, and this often leads to mistakes and lack of judgment, which can get them into trouble. Adolescents are usually very aware of the need to conform to the norms of their peer group and may be preoccupied with how they look, what clothes they are wearing, and how popular they are. Adolescence can be a very difficult time if the young man thinks and feels that he is different. If his peers see him as being different, he may be isolated, teased, and ridiculed, and this can have lifelong consequences, with low self-esteem as the usual result. Low self-esteem can lead to risky social and sexual activities, as well as feelings of inadequacy that influence occupational and relationship choices.

But most young men negotiate this passage into adulthood just fine. Somewhere along the way, they discover who they are attracted to and usually act on that attraction. Young men who are attracted to women often have their hearts broken many times on the road to a lasting relationship. Those who are attracted to men must negotiate a world of stigma and marginalization where homosexual attraction is still seen as different and not legitimate. Confusion about sexual attraction is common during adolescence, but the negative societal messages about same-sex attraction further compound the issue.

The major tasks of adolescence that must be accomplished before adulthood are separation from family and achievement of independence, as well as finding a vocational goal. The adolescent must be able to control his impulses and deal with frustration in a constructive way, and he must also learn to delay gratification of his wishes. And to round out this challenging list of tasks, the adolescent must develop a healthy and realistic sense of self and reach a mature level of sexuality.

Most young men masturbate, and this solitary sexual activity usually persists into adulthood. Even though it is universally practiced, many young men feel guilty about this, and in parts of our society it is still a taboo topic, and not much is said about it by parents or other adult authorities. Some religious and cultural institutions still frown upon masturbation, and many young men struggle with the drive to do it, the pleasure that results from it, and the subsequent feelings of shame and guilt.

Young men often feel pressure to become sexually active. There is a great deal of boasting about sexual experience among young men, and the facts are often quite different from what they tell their friends. This persists into adulthood where men often don't speak honestly about sex—their feelings and experiences—but rather inflate their stories and never talk about their true emotions. Young men also receive conflicting messages about sex: "Get all you can" versus "Don't take advantage," or "Sex is the greatest" versus "Don't get into trouble." Much of the information that appears in the media is also contradictory. On the one hand, sex is shown as something that is highly pleasurable, and those who have sex are cool and manly, but on the other hand, sex is also dangerous, as it leads to sexually transmitted infections and pregnancy. Adolescents commonly are thought of as viewing themselves as immortal, invulnerable, and immune and are treated accordingly by their parents and teachers. Therefore, the messages they receive are about preventing themselves from getting into trouble and not about how to be a sexually healthy young person.

When an adolescent gets cancer, everything changes. The young man may be more dependent on his parents for help with activities of daily living; this may lead to an inability to achieve the developmental task of independence. The adolescent may miss extended periods of school, and the social consequences of that may affect his ability to make and keep peer relationships in the future. Treatment for cancer may cause physical changes, and for a young person who is trying to look like everyone else, this can be a significant challenge. He may avoid social situations because he is embarrassed by scars from surgery, weight gain or loss from chemotherapy, or other side effects of medications or radiation therapy. Some treatments interfere with normal growth and development, including sexual development, so the young man may look many years younger than he really is.

In short, a life-threatening illness like cancer challenges the notion of adolescents as immortal, invulnerable, and immune. However, 80% of children and adolescents treated for cancer now survive the disease and grow into adulthood.

But their lives are fundamentally changed by the disease and the experience. Some may be infertile, which may affect their decision to enter a permanent relationship in adulthood. On the other hand, others may assume that they are infertile and so may not use contraception and then go on to father children when they don't want to or with the wrong person.

Young Adulthood

Young adulthood is the period between ages 20 and 40 and is a time of great social and emotional growth. Physical growth does not really occur at this time; however, some young men do gain some height in their early 20s. In these two decades, most people decide whether to get married and whether to parent. This is also a time when many men build their careers or at least settle down in a career for the future. Cancer in this period presents some unique challenges.

One of the most significant challenges for men who have had cancer is how to tell a new or prospective partner that they have had cancer, that they may not be able to father children, or that they are missing a body part, or have an ostomy bag, or many scars. When do you tell someone, and what do you do if that person rejects you? For the man who is partnered when the diagnosis of cancer is made, this relationship usually proves to be a source of strength and comfort. Most couples report that the cancer experience brought them closer and enhanced their commitment and the depth of their emotions for each other.

A young adult dealing with cancer or its aftermath may have a very different attitude toward life compared to his peers. He may be more serious or perhaps a greater risk taker. The cancer treatments will affect him not only physically but also emotionally and socially, and he may have to delay some of the important tasks of young adulthood, such as establishing a career, because of extended periods in the hospital or time spent recuperating from chemotherapy. This can also affect his ability to form romantic relationships and to establish a strong social peer group. The illness may mean that the man has to remain in his parents' home instead of moving out, and he may be physically and financially dependent on them far beyond the time his peers move out and make their own way in the world.

Fertility issues usually become important for men in these decades, although some men may wish to start their family when they are past 40 years of age. For the childhood cancer survivor who reaches young adulthood, this may be the first time that he has to deal with this issue. When cancer is diagnosed in childhood, decisions about treatment usually are made in a great hurry, and most parents are concerned only about the survival of their precious child. Delaying treatment to think about fertility far in the future is not something that most would even consider. But the treatment may render the young man infertile, and it is in young adulthood that this is discovered. Some men may be angry that nothing was done to preserve their fertility back then or that no attempts were made to freeze sperm. This is, of course, dependent on the sexual development of the child in the past, as development of sperm occurs during puberty; so, if the cancer occurred in early childhood, nothing can be done. But the man may not understand this and may be regretful about decisions that he was not part of in the distant past.

Middle Adulthood

Middle adulthood covers the years from age 40 to about age 65. This is usually a time of secure primary relationships, well-established careers winding down into retirement, and parenting responsibilities becoming less intense as children grow and form their own families. Ill health is more common during this period, and men in this age group may experience medical diseases such as high blood pressure, raised cholesterol, and diabetes. The later years of middle adulthood are also the years when a diagnosis of cancer is most common.

This is also the period when some men notice that their sexual functioning changes. The most common challenge to men in these years is the onset of some difficulties with achieving and maintaining erections. This may be linked to the onset of cardiac disease or diabetes and often causes distress to the man and his partner. During this same time, the female partner of the man may be going through the menopausal transition, and her sexual interest may wane, causing more or less distress to the couple. Some men also notice a decline in their level of sexual desire coupled with a change in body fat and loss of muscle mass. This is probably caused by slowly declining levels of testosterone but may also be associated with decreased physical activity.

The focus of society is on youth and strength, and loss of both in combination with ill health may affect the man not only physically but also in the way he sees himself as a man and a member of society. This can be a time when the losses associated with cancer cause significant challenges for the man. Loss of a partner to cancer means that the older man may be seeking social and emotional support at a time when he is not confident in his ability to attract someone new. He may not want to feel like a burden to his adult children, and he may be lonely.

Older Adulthood

Older adulthood is a time when physical changes are inevitable. However, they do not necessarily mean the end of vibrancy and enjoyment of life. It is also a time when illness and disability are more common, and the loss of friends and one's partner is a reality.

In our youth-obsessed culture, it is often assumed that older adults, those age 65 and older, are not sexual. In fact, this is one of the last social taboos that we hardly talk about. However, recent surveys suggest that partnered older adults continue to enjoy regular sexual activity that they find satisfying. Older adults have the same needs for physical and emotional love and support, and many will seek new relationships after the loss of a long-term partner or spouse to avoid the loneliness of being single in their later years.

The Words We Use

With all this talk about sex, sex, sex, it is important to understand the difference between some of the terms used throughout this book and in our daily conversations about this important topic. The two major terms are *sexuality* and *sexual functioning*. *Sexuality* means how we express and experience ourselves as sexual beings. This is a lifelong process that begins in infancy and remains a vital part of our lives until death. It encompasses our image of ourselves as men (and women) and how we interact with others of both sexes, and is essentially a process that takes place in our brains. Sexuality is influenced by the messages we received from our family as children and from our peers and society as a whole. Our sexuality encompasses our sexual orientation and where and how we seek sexual pleasure. It is strongly influenced by religion, culture, and ethnicity, as well as education and experience. It is not a rational process but rather an innate characteristic. And our expression of sexuality is not dependent on being in a relationship; as single and partnered individuals, our sexuality is a unique part of ourselves.

On the other hand, *sexual functioning* is what we *do* as sexual beings. Sexual behavior is something that is learned over the years. This learning is influenced by experimentation with what feels good for our own bodies and what brings pleasure to others when we touch them. Curiosity leads to further experimentation, and pleasure reinforces these activities. However, social taboos and restrictions seek to limit what is regarded as normal and healthy, and this is something that changes over time. As such, it should be viewed within the context of history, culture, and time. There has always been wide variation in sexual practice across societies, cultures, and geography; no single one is right or wrong, acceptable or deviant.

Most of us have our own language for what we think and do regarding sexuality and sexual activity. We even have our own language for our body parts, and men are much more likely than women to have an affectionate name for their genitals. This may have something to do with comfort as well as the visibility of the male genitalia. Some of the language used with regard to sexual activity tends to be euphemistic (for example, describing sexual intercourse as *intimacy* instead of using the word *sex*). Sexual activity itself has many meanings: It may describe sexual intercourse, oral sex, or masturbation alone or with a partner. This can cause all kinds of confusion when trying to explain what you want or what you did, or what you don't want to do! Euphemisms tend to make us feel more comfortable but can obviously lead to problems when the meanings aren't clear.

Our sexual behaviors may change over time and under the influence of many different factors in our lives. Being partnered for some men means having regular sex, while for others it may mean having less sex than when they were single. Sex may be more or less important at different stages of our lives and for many different reasons. Male sexuality also contains many myths, many of which men believe themselves. A good example of this is that male sexuality is simple, like a light switch. Men are either turned on or not, and it is easy to get turned on under any circumstances.

In fact, male sexuality is a complex phenomenon comprising biologic factors (the body, sexual drive, erectile capacity and ejaculation, and sexual satisfaction), and these are under the influence of hormones and blood and nerve supply, as well as personal health behaviors. A second factor is that of psychological influences (cognition [thoughts], behaviors, and emotions). A relationship dimension also exists that reflects the man's way of interacting with a partner and how he is able to empathize and support the partner. Societal norms play a role in how men react and interact. And finally, psychosexual skills (one's sexual response and knowledge) are an integral part of a man's sexuality and sexual life. No simple light switch there!

Sexuality and Cancer

For many people, these two words just don't go together. For many years, talking about cancer was a big taboo, and at the same time, sex was not discussed either. Both were secretive subjects that were talked about in private, if discussed at all. Things are different now: Cancer is seen in a different light, and we are much more open about sex. Sex and cancer can and do go together, because cancer is beatable and sex is part of life. According to the American Cancer Society, at least 10.5 million Americans with a history of cancer were alive in 2003, and between 1996 and 2002, survival rates were up 51% over previous decades. People with cancer are living longer and better. They are returning to work and social life, and they and their partners continue to have sexual wants and needs. Quality of life after cancer has become an important part of how we view the success (or failure) of cancer treatment. And sexuality is an important part of quality of life affecting physical and emotional aspects.

The site of the cancer may have a lot to do with the sexual consequences of both the cancer and its treatments. For example, a man with prostate cancer will be expected to have some problems with erections following both surgery and radiation because the erectile nerves are found on the outside of the prostate gland. But with other cancers, the sexual consequences are not that clear and may be much more subtle. For example, surgery for cancer may leave a man with a large scar on his body. How this affects his body image can affect how he sees himself as a sexual being. The man with a colostomy bag may feel sexually unattractive and may avoid his partner out of fear of being rejected. His partner, in turn, feels rejected because the man no longer seems to want contact with him or her. This book describes in detail what these changes are and how they can affect the individual and his partner.

The stages of the cancer experience also play a role in when and how sexuality is affected. The time of diagnosis usually is one of crisis and anxiety. The person has to undergo many different tests, and there sometimes are extended periods of waiting for test results and doctor's appointments. All of this causes uncertainty, and human beings usually don't do well with uncertainty; we prefer to *know* what is happening. Once we know that it is cancer, life is never the same again. For most people, a diagnosis of cancer presents a life-threatening challenge. Everything is thrown into chaos: Will I live? What will happen to my family? How bad are the treatments going to be? Am I going to make it? How this affects sexuality and sexual functioning is as different as people are different. Some men find that during this period, their desire for sex disappears. They don't think about it and don't seem to care about it. This is a natural reaction to an extremely stressful event. Others seem more interested in sex and may be more demanding of their partner or masturbate more. This is also a normal reaction because sex brings comfort and pleasure and is a great way to distract oneself from the harsh reality of a new diagnosis. It is also a way of connecting with one's partner and seeking support and love. Many people report that at this time sex takes on a new meaning and brings with it a poignancy and sense of pleasure unique to the couple.

The period when treatment takes place can stretch over many weeks or months. The most common treatments for cancer—surgery, radiation, and chemotherapy—may be given alone or in some combination. Every year new treatments become available, such as immunotherapy and agents that prevent blood from reaching tumors. All of these can affect sexuality in one way or another. Cancer treatment can alter levels of hormones and can disrupt nerve and blood supply to sexual and adjacent organs. The treatment can also affect mood and how we see ourselves as sexual beings. These changes may be temporary or may last for many years after treatment.

The active treatment phase is usually one where sexual activity is not a priority for the patient, but everyone is different. For some men, being sexual in the face of disease is one way of showing the cancer who's the boss and refusing to give in. For others, the side effects of treatment (such as nausea, pain, fatigue, and dizziness) preclude even the thought of anything sexual being possible. And still others want to experience the pleasure that sexual activity brings as a way of comforting themselves and their partner. There really is no right or wrong way to be during treatment.

But one day, the treatment will be over, and the person moves into the more chronic stage of the illness. This is an extended period of time when life begins to go back to normal, but thoughts of the cancer and fear of recurrence are common. Many people regard this phase as the survivorship phase, and some say that once you have had cancer, you are forever changed and are, from that time on, a cancer survivor. Others don't like the term and prefer to put the cancer behind them and try not to think about it. It is often in this stage when couples resume sexual activity, and so it is during this time that they notice something is not as it used to be. Men may notice that things are different in the quality of their erections independent of sexual activity or may notice that they no longer have erections upon wakening in the morning. They may also notice changes when masturbating, which can affect when and if they try to resume partnered sexual activity. Some men experience little or no disruption in their sexual lives, and some report that after getting through the treatment, sex is even better than before because they are more in touch with their bodies and want to embrace life with a new intensity. Once again, any and all of these experiences are perfectly normal.

Talking About It

Although men often laugh and joke about sex, having a serious conversation about it is something else. Most of us have some difficulty finding the right words to say when it comes to this topic. And it is particularly difficult to talk to healthcare providers about this. Often the appointment is rushed and you only have the opportunity to ask when the doctor has his hand on the door and asks you if there is anything else you'd like to talk about. (This is called the *doorknob syndrome* and is recognized as a barrier to communication.)

Research has shown that healthcare providers are willing to talk about sexual issues with patients if the patient brings it up. And the same research shows that patients wait for the healthcare provider to ask about it. The result is silence, with both parties waiting for the other to go first. The reasons why this happens are similar for both patient and provider: embarrassment and not wanting to ask about or discuss a private part of life. There are some differences, however. Many healthcare providers have received very little education about human sexuality and are afraid of being seen as lacking knowledge on the subject if the patient asks. At the same time, some patients are afraid that they will seem stupid for asking a question. Some healthcare providers think that it is someone else's responsibility and that their primary goal is to cure the cancer and leave all the other "stuff" to someone else, whoever that may be. And patients may not know who to ask, because no one on the healthcare team has ever asked if they have any concerns or questions. What a mess!

It can also be difficult for one man to talk to another man about sexual difficulties. This may represent some sort of symbolic weakness and may also be why men tend to joke about sex a lot. Your healthcare provider may be much older or much younger than you, and age can sometimes present a significant barrier. Young people find it difficult to talk to older people about sex (because older people aren't having it and don't know anything about it!) and vice versa.

That is why I wrote this book. I believe that all people—man or woman, young or old, partnered or single, gay or straight—have the right to ask questions about sexuality and sexual functioning and to have those questions answered in a way that they understand and that makes sense to them. I have done this in three different ways. First, I wrote a textbook for healthcare professionals called *Breaking the Silence on Cancer and Sexuality: A Handbook for Healthcare Providers*. This book provides a comprehensive overview of cancer and the sexual consequences of treatment. Then, I wrote a book for women with cancer called *Woman Cancer Sex*. And now there is this book for men and the women and men who love them.

What Can You Expect From This Book?

This book is divided into three parts. This chapter and the one following provide some basic information about how things work and why. This is important information and shouldn't be skipped over, because understanding this forms the basis of understanding how cancer affects sexuality.

The second section of the book contains the stories of 10 men, all of whom have or have had cancer. Each man experiences some sort of sexual difficulty, and his story is told in the chapter, along with explanations and suggestions for how to get help or help yourself. The chapters cover everything from loss of interest in sex to changes in body image, problems with erections, and pain with orgasm. There is a chapter about what happens to the partner of a man with cancer. It is important to read all these chapters even if you don't have the same kind of cancer. There is information in each chapter that will be of interest and use to you, no matter what kind of cancer you had or how long ago it was, or if you are older or younger than the man whose story is told in the chapter. And ask your partner to read it too. Or, if you don't have a partner now, sometime in the future this book may help a new partner understand some of what you went through or may still be dealing with.

The final part of the book has two chapters. One addresses the important topic of communication with your partner, and the very last chapter has useful resources to help you find your way to additional help and information.

Most people diagnosed with cancer today will go on to live for many years, hopefully with good quality of life. And sexuality is a part of that quality of life. This book was written to help you access the information and tools to reclaim sexual health after the fight for life has been won.

CHAPTER 2

How Do Things Work?

We know that cancer affects sexuality and sexual functioning. In men, we often see direct effects on different aspects of sexual activity. To understand this more fully, it is important to know the range of normal male sexual functioning. To do that, one needs to understand both the anatomy (the parts) and the physiology (the actions) of the male sexual organs, as well as the thoughts, feelings, and values of the man with those parts. This chapter describes male sexual anatomy and what the different parts do during the different phases of sexual activity. It also presents information about what we know regarding how men behave during sexual encounters.

Male Sexual Anatomy

The male sexual organs are easy to find, as they are mostly external. The penis and the scrotum lie outside the body. The penis is composed of three cylinders of spongy tissue that lie along the length of the penis. Two of these cylinders are known as the spongy tissues or corpora cavernosa, and these fill with blood during an erection. The other cylinder (the corpus spongiosum) surrounds the urethra, the tube through which urine and semen pass. The end of the penis is called the glans, and at birth it is covered by tissue called the foreskin. Some parents choose to have this foreskin surgically removed when their baby boy is just a few days old; this is called circumcision.

The scrotum is covered in hair after puberty and contains two testicles, which produce an important hormone, testosterone, as well as sperm. The sperm leave the testicles via two long tubes, the vas deferens, and travel to the prostate. In the prostate, fluid from the seminal vesicles (two small glands located slightly above the prostate) joins the sperm, and during orgasm this seminal fluid is pushed to the outside through the urethra as part of orgasm.

The prostate gland lies under the bladder and is about the size of a walnut. The purpose of this gland is to make fluid that is part of the ejaculate. Two tiny glands called Cowper's glands (bulbourethral glands) lie below the prostate gland. The fluid from these glands is often seen as a small drop at the tip of the penis during arousal.

Two structures in the brain are important for sexual functioning because of the role they play in the production of hormones. The hypothalamus and the pituitary gland regulate production of testosterone by the testicles and to a much lesser extent by the adrenal glands that lie on top of the kidneys. Testosterone production at puberty is responsible for the typical male characteristics, such as body hair, broadening of the shoulders, growth of facial hair, and growth of the larynx (voice box) that causes deepening of the voice as well as sexual drive, thoughts, and fantasies. Men have low levels of estrogen in their bodies, as well. Another hormone, prolactin, is responsible, in part, for the control of testosterone levels in the bloodstream.

The Sexual Response Cycle

It is often said that the brain is the biggest sex organ. This is true in that the brain has an important function not just in regulating the production of hormones but also because it is in the brain that we experience sexual thoughts and fantasies as well as interpreting touch as sexual and determining whether it is pleasurable or not. In response, the brain also sends signals to the genital organs causing the typical signs and sensations of arousal.

Since the 1960s, we have had some understanding of how humans react as sexual beings. This is in large part because of the work of the famous sexologists William Masters and Virginia Johnson. Based on their observations of people in the laboratory, they developed a four-stage model that has become the cornerstone of our understanding of this phenomenon and has influenced many other sex researchers.

Masters and Johnson's model describes four phases that are linear (one follows another) and very similar for men and women. The four stages of their model are excitement, plateau, orgasm, and resolution. These represent episodes of swelling caused by increased blood flow as well as muscular contractions.

In the first stage, the excitement stage, heart rate and blood pressure increase and blood flows into the tissues of the sexual organs. The penis becomes erect and enlarges as blood flows into the spongy tissues. The skin of the scrotum thickens, and the testicles grow bigger. The scrotum elevates and moves in toward the body.

The second stage, the plateau, is essentially a state of advanced arousal. Blood pressure and heart rate continue to increase, and breathing becomes rapid. Some people have involuntary facial grimaces, and the hands and feet may contract. The testicles continue to enlarge and move into the body. The head of the penis changes to a deeper color because of the increased amount of blood in the area. The Cowper's glands secrete some fluid that can be seen at the tip of the penis.

The next stage, orgasm, is the one when intense pleasure is felt, in part because of muscular contractions. Respiration and heart rate peak as feelings of intense pleasure radiate throughout the body. The muscles of the pelvic floor, the anal sphincter, and major muscles of the arms and legs contract and sometimes even go into spasm. For most men, orgasm is the time when ejaculation occurs. During the first part of ejaculation, fluid is pushed toward the penis by contractions of the prostate gland and the vas deferens. The entrance to the bladder closes to prevent mixing of semen and urine in the bladder. When this fluid enters the penis, men experience a sensation called *ejaculatory inevitability*; most men are unable to stop their orgasm at this point. In the second part of ejaculation, the fluid is propelled along the urethra and out of the penis.

The final stage, resolution, describes the process of blood flowing out of the tissues and heart rate, blood pressure, and respirations returning to normal. The penis loses rigidity in two phases: First, blood flows out of the spongy bodies, and then out of the corpus spongiosum around the urethra. The scrotum and testicles also return to their usual size. In men, orgasm is followed by a period, the refractory period, where they cannot have another erection or orgasm. How long this lasts is largely age dependent. In young men, this stage may last only a few minutes. In older men, it may last hours or even days.

Almost 20 years later, a student of Masters and Johnson refined their model and introduced the idea of sexual desire. Helen Singer Kaplan described the sexual response cycle as having three parts: desire, excitement, and orgasm. Kaplan saw desire as part emotion and part cognition. In Kaplan's model, excitement is much like that described by Masters and Johnson, with swelling of genital tissues in response to an increase in blood flow. The final phase in her model is that of orgasm, which she described as a series of muscle contractions. Although Kaplan did not see her model as being linear with one stage following the next, many have interpreted it that way.

A five-stage model has been proposed by Zilbergeld and Ellison. Their model comprises the following phases: interest, arousal, physiologic readiness, orgasm, and satisfaction. *Interest* in this model is essentially the same as *desire* in Kaplan's model. Arousal is a physiologic process in which blood flows into the penis and scrotum. In this model, readiness is described as an erection sufficient for penetration. Orgasm is like the other models described previously, but Zilbergeld and Ellison described this stage as having two parts: the muscle contractions and the physical sensations. The last stage of their model, satisfaction, refers to a subjective cognitive and emotional appraisal of the experience.

Sexual Behavior in Humans

How do we know how to behave as sexual beings? Is this an instinctive or a learned behavior? Why do we do the things we do in a sexual encounter? The answers to these questions are answered, in part, by the idea of sexual scripts. Sexual scripts are the learned behaviors, feelings, and meanings that we attach to sexual behavior. Every man (and woman) has learned over time what attracts them, what feels good, and how they approach sexual experiences.

For many men, their first sexual experiences are solitary and may begin in the womb. Medical and nursing personnel have observed male fetuses playing with their penises even before birth. Whether this touching is pleasurable is not something that can be determined. But many male babies will play with their genitals if they get the chance; often when their diaper is removed, their hands make a beeline to the penis! Babies also are able to have erections; many mothers will say that their infant sons appear to be having fun when touching themselves. Across the life span, boys and men engage in masturbation frequently and consistently.

Men's sexual behavior also is influenced by messages from peers and the media. The media generally portray men as sexual initiators and also as always ready, willing, and able. A great deal of peer pressure exists for young men to gain sexual experience, and they often are expected to share tales of their sexual exploits within the peer group. For men who are not sexually experienced or who are consciously delaying sexual activity, this peer pressure can be relentless and upsetting.

Men and women develop sexual scripts, especially when they are a couple. These sexual scripts dictate what happens during sexual activity. For example, some couples always have sex on a Saturday night, at 10:30 with the lights off. This is a routine, and what happens during the sexual encounter may never deviate from a set of activities. Ten minutes of kissing and touching the genitals, and then the man lies on top of the woman and inserts his penis into her vagina. After three to four minutes of thrusting, he has an orgasm and moves to his side of the bed and goes to sleep. Other couples may have more adventurous or experimental sexual scripts that may involve fantasy, dressing up, watching suggestive videos, or trying different positions for sex. One sexual script is not right or better than another. If both partners are happy and satisfied with their sexual script (or scripts), then everything is fine.

People tend to use the same script over and over as that script tends to be reinforced by positive rewards. When the individual or couple is challenged by cancer that temporarily or permanently changes the anatomy of the sexual organs or interferes with sexual feelings, this may necessitate a change to their usual sexual script. The result may be that the individual or couple is not able to change and sexual activity may cease, or the partners may be able to adapt with a new script and continue a healthy sexual relationship.

Conclusion

This chapter has described how male sexual anatomy is structured and how sexologists have described the way they work. But male sexuality is far more complex than just a penis that gets hard or not. Emotions and thoughts play a large role in male sexual functioning, even though men are often depicted as being sexual robots who can and do perform under even the most challenging environments. In the following chapters, you will read the stories of men with different kinds of cancer who are challenged in this intimate part of their lives and who struggle with sexual and emotional difficulties as a result of the cancer and/or its treatment.

PART TWO

What Happened?
Cancer and Sex

In this section you will meet 10 different men and their partners. All these men have had some kind of cancer, and all have experienced some kind of sexual difficulty as a result of the cancer and/or its treatment.

You will have an intimate view of their lives and struggles, as well as explanations of why they are experiencing sexual problems and how they overcame them or adapted to them.

The explanations by Dr. Katz are followed by tips that can help you as you try to deal with the same kinds of issues. Take-Away Points provide real and useful information for sexual and treatment-related problems.

CHAPTER 3

Loss of Libido

Sex never even enters my mind anymore.

Loss of libido is a common complaint of people with cancer. Nowhere is this more apparent than for men on androgen deprivation therapy for the treatment of advanced prostate cancer. Testosterone plays an important role in the experience of libido, and when men are on androgen deprivation therapy, their levels of testosterone drop rapidly. This usually results in an absence of the sense of sexual desire, which can affect the man beyond his primary emotional relationship. For many men, this desire has been an important aspect of their daily lives. Some men are only aware of the usual presence of this desire when they notice that it is gone.

In this chapter, you will meet Ted, a 61-year-old man who has been on androgen deprivation therapy for almost two years. Ted has advanced prostate cancer, and this treatment has been ordered because when he was diagnosed, the cancer had already spread to his bones. Ted is mourning not only the state of his cancer but also the changes brought on by the lack of testosterone in his body.

At the end of this chapter, you will understand

- The treatment for advanced prostate cancer
- The effects of androgen therapy on a man's sexual desire
- Other effects of androgen deprivation therapy.

Ted's Story

Like many men his age, Ted has been having his prostate-specific antigen (PSA) measured every year when he has his physical. Over the past three years it had been going up slowly, but from last year to this year it had almost tripled. His family physician did not seem very worried but referred Ted to a urologist. The urologist reviewed Ted's PSA results from the past 10 years and indicated that he was concerned about the big jump over the past year. He suggested that Ted have a prostate biopsy immediately. The biopsy was performed the next week by the urologist. During the procedure, he told Ted that his prostate felt abnormal and that this was concerning. Two weeks after the biopsy, Ted received a call from the urologist. As the doctor suspected, the biopsy showed that Ted had prostate cancer, and the urologist asked him to come in to discuss his treatment options.

Ted went to the appointment alone; his wife, Joan, was having some health issues of her own, and he didn't want to bother her. In fact, he hadn't told her anything about what was going on, not even that he'd had the prostate biopsy. They had been married for just over 35 years, and she was the light of his life. They had one child, Barry, who lived in Houston, where he worked for NASA. They were so proud of their "rocket scientist" and the success he had made of his life. They were also the proud grandparents of Teddy, a seven-year-old named for his grandfather who had the energy of a hummingbird.

The waiting room at the urologist's office was very full, and Ted's appointment time came and went. He grew increasingly irritated as the minutes ticked by. No one told the waiting patients why they had not been seen, and no one had been called to see the doctor for at least 45 minutes. After waiting for almost two hours, Ted left the waiting room and went home. What was the big deal? He was feeling fine and had no symptoms at all. Soon he had almost forgotten about the biopsy. No one called him, and so he decided there was nothing to worry about.

But nine months later, he noticed that his right hip was painful. At first he put it down to a muscle sprain—he had been cleaning out the garage and perhaps had overdone things. But the pain didn't go away, and so he made an appointment to see his family physician, Dr. Bryant. Prior to seeing Ted, the doctor reviewed his chart. He read the letter from the urologist that reported on Ted's biopsy results and was shocked to realize that it appeared Ted had never had any treatment for his prostate cancer. The cancer was advanced when it was diagnosed more than nine months ago!

The appointment did not go as Ted thought it would. Dr. Bryant's face was very serious as he explained to Ted that according to the biopsy results, he had advanced prostate cancer. The doctor was also concerned that the hip pain Ted had noticed may be more than a strain. Dr. Bryant had called the urologist and arranged for Ted to see him later the same day.

Dr. Katz Explains

Since the introduction of the PSA test more than 20 years ago, most men are now diagnosed with early, localized prostate cancer. The PSA test is a blood test that measures the level of a protein that is produced by the prostate gland itself as well as by prostate cancer cells. It is a screening test, and the definitive test for prostate cancer is a biopsy, in which 12 or more samples are taken in a planned manner from all areas of the prostate. A pathologist examines the samples of prostate tissue under a microscope, and if cancerous cells are present, the grade of the cancer and its aggressiveness are determined. This is called the Gleason score and ranges from 6 to 10. Additional information is also provided by what the doctor feels when he examines the prostate by doing a digital rectal exam (known as DRE).

Many men do not have any symptoms when they have prostate cancer, especially if it is in the early stages. When the cancer is more advanced, it may spread to the lymph nodes and also to the bones. Pain in the bones, particularly in the pelvic and hip area, is concerning and should never be ignored. It may be a muscle strain, but it may also be something more serious.

Not Good News

This time when Ted went to the urologist's office, the waiting room was much less busy. He waited just a few minutes before being called into the doctor's office. The urologist was matter of fact: Ted's cancer was advanced nine months ago when he had the biopsy. He was going to need additional testing to determine exactly what the situation was now, and the tests needed to be done immediately. Ted didn't ask many questions; he felt embarrassed that he had ignored this and was very frightened. That afternoon he had another biopsy of his prostate gland and a blood test, and the next day he was scheduled for a bone scan.

When he got home, he told Joan everything. It was a relief to admit to someone how stupid he felt. Joan was shocked and more than a little angry that he had not told her anything. In her usual pragmatic way, she told him that he needed to find out exactly where things stood, and she was going to make sure he never missed another appointment.

The bone scan went well, and he was told to contact his physician for the results. By the time he got home, there was a message from the urologist's office for him to come in at the end of the week to review the test results. This time he planned to take Joan with him.

Dr. Katz Explains

Because nine months had passed since his first biopsy, the urologist wanted to repeat the biopsy to make sure that he had accurate information about what was happening inside Ted's body. The bone scan was performed to determine whether there had been spread outside the prostate and to the bones. A bone scan is not usually done when the biopsy indicates that the cancer is still in the early stages, but when the cancer is more advanced, it is important to know this, as the treatment of the cancer will be different.

It is always a good idea to take someone with you when you go to a medical appointment. It is especially important when you expect to hear the results of tests and if there is concern that the results may indicate cancer. Most people don't hear much after they've heard the words "you have cancer," and having a second pair of ears there can be very useful. The person with you may be able to take notes, and this is also helpful when you want to review what was said at the appointment. You may have different recollections about what was said, and the notes will be more accurate than your memories.

The Plan

Ted could tell that Joan was very nervous when they reached the urologist's office. He felt strangely calm, but then he had known about this for many months.

It was all new to Joan. His embarrassment had now turned to guilt, and he felt bad that he had not told Joan at the time. It was difficult to see how upset she was, and he was responsible for this.

After a brief wait, they were called into the urologist's office. Once again the specialist was matter of fact: Ted had advanced prostate cancer that had spread to his bones; the pain he felt in his hip was a result of this spread. Because the cancer was advanced, surgery or radiation would not be used to treat the cancer. He was going to have to take medication to starve the cancer of testosterone.

Ted could sense Joan's reaction to this information; he could not bring himself to look at her but he felt her body tense and her hands start to shake. She started to ask a question but the urologist interrupted her. "My nurse will explain all of the details. You need to take some pills, and we will give you an injection today. I will see you every three months from now on." And with that he ushered them out of his office and into an examination room.

The nurse knocked on the door within minutes. Ted had still not said anything, and Joan was crying softly. This was such a shock for her, and he wanted to comfort her but was afraid he would lose control, and how could he help her then? The nurse entered the room and immediately offered Joan a box of tissues. She sat quietly while Joan sniffled, blew her nose, and dried her tears. For the next 10 minutes the nurse explained what would come next. She spoke softly, and her calm manner seemed to help Joan. Ted's mind was racing; what did all of this mean, and how had this happened to him? The nurse explained that Ted would need to take some pills for a month to block the effect of testosterone in his body. She was also going to give him an injection today that would last for three months. He would need to come back every three months and they would monitor his PSA levels to see if they dropped.

The nurse's voice and calm manner helped Ted to calm his thoughts. He had to ask her to repeat some things, but as they talked, he realized that now he had a plan. He took the prescription from her and made a mental note to stop at the drugstore on the way home. Then she talked for a while about the side effects of the injection, and his mind started wandering again. Joan was listening attentively, so he just sat back and let his thoughts go. The nurse gave him the injection and it hurt a bit, but at least they had a plan.

Dr. Katz Explains

When prostate cancer is more advanced, such as in Ted's case, treating the prostate with radiation or surgery will not be effective. When the cancer has spread outside the prostate, the most effective way to treat it is to starve it by removing testosterone from the body. There are two ways to do this. One way is to surgically remove the man's testicles, called surgical castration. This used to be the only way to remove testosterone from a man's body. About 20 years ago, medications were developed that interrupt the signal from the brain to the testicles to produce the hormone. These medications are called luteinizing hormone–releasing hormone agonists and are given by injection every one to six months. Some people call this regimen of medications "hormone therapy," but that does not accurately represent what the medications are given for. A more accurate term is *androgen deprivation therapy* because the medications deprive the body and the cancer of the male hormone testosterone, which is also known as an androgen.

Initially, the brain responds to the low levels of testosterone by instructing the testicles to produce more testosterone; this is called a *flare*. To prevent it, many doctors prescribe pills called nonsteroidal antiandrogens for the first few weeks of treatment. This medication prevents the cancer cells from absorbing the additional testosterone produced by the flare. Men whose cancer has spread to the bones, as in Ted's case, find that the medication helps to reduce the pain they experience in their bones.

Did Someone Mention Side Effects?

Ted returned home after the appointment feeling better than he did when they set out to see the urologist. It felt like they had a plan. Joan was very quiet, and Ted was a little afraid to ask her what was wrong. He knew this was a shock to her, and he felt really bad that he hadn't told her about this from the beginning. But they had a plan! It was going to be okay.

He'd remembered to stop at the drugstore to fill the prescription for the pills the doctor had prescribed, and the bottle was sitting on the kitchen table. The pharmacist had wanted to spend some time with him explaining about the pills, but Ted wanted to get home and so had declined to have the talk. He just wanted to get on with things. Joan did not talk much at dinner, and he left her to her thoughts; it was better this way. When she wanted to say something, she would. They went to bed in silence. As he lay in the dark, Ted couldn't remember the last time this had happened. They usually talked for a while before turning out the light.

Ted eventually fell asleep but was woken a few hours later by a sensation that he had never experienced before. It was as if someone had thrown a pail of hot water over him. He sat up in bed, gasping for air. His T-shirt was soaking wet, and he felt like his skin was on fire. What was happening? The sweating stopped in a few minutes, and then he felt so cold. He started to shiver as his wet clothes cooled down. Joan turned over, aware even in her sleep that something was wrong. "It's the hot flashes the nurse warned you about," she mumbled. "Were you not listening?"

Then he remembered. The nurse had mentioned something about hot flashes, but that was the part that he didn't really want to hear. What else had she talked about? He got out of bed and went to find a dry T-shirt to wear. When he came back to bed he noticed that the sheets on his side of the bed were wet and cold. Joan was deeply asleep, so he went downstairs to the TV room, covered himself with a throw, and fell asleep on the sofa.

Dr. Katz Explains

Hot flashes are a common side effect of these medications. They can happen at any time of the day or night. They often feel like a wave of heat traveling through the body and usually are accompanied by sweating. Some men notice that their face, neck, and chest turn red at the same time. When they happen at night, the sweating may be more noticeable, and they are then called night sweats.

Take-Away Points

- Many men find that wearing lighter clothes helps reduce sweating.
- Having a ceiling fan in the bedroom may help when a hot flash occurs during the night, but when the sweating stops, you need to turn off the fan to prevent the chills.
- Layering some towels on the bed also may help; when one gets wet, you can take it off and return to sleeping without having to change the bedsheets.
- Medication can help control hot flashes; speak to your physician if the hot flashes are severe.

Body Changes

Ted got used to the hot flashes. He even managed to laugh a bit when Joan reminded him about how she suffered when she was going through menopause. He noticed that the pain in his hip had gone away completely, and he was happy about this. He had always been a very active person, and since taking early retirement, he enjoyed having more time to hike in the mountains and play golf in the summer. But he was too tired these days, and this was frustrating. He just felt tired all the time and not like himself at all.

It had been five weeks since he had the injection. He'd gained six pounds in the last month and felt as though his body was becoming soft. When he looked in the mirror he just didn't look the same. The hot flashes were worse at night, and he was pretty grumpy because he was not sleeping well. He spent most nights in the TV room; he didn't want to disturb Joan's sleep and he found it really difficult to go back to sleep after a hot flash woke him. So he slept on the sofa. It wasn't perfect, and Joan complained that she missed him at night.

But something else bothered him even more than the hot flashes. He had not touched Joan since the day he had his first injection. He hadn't noticed that things were different, but she did, and she complained about it. They had always had a very affectionate relationship. Their friends teased them about it. And it was true; after 35 years of marriage they still held hands when they went for a walk, and they kissed each other frequently during the day. Sure, things had slowed down in the bed department, but he still liked to touch her, especially when she wasn't expecting it. But since that injection, he hadn't thought about anything sexual at all. Only when Joan told him that he'd stopped kissing and touching her did he realize that it was true.

Dr. Katz Explains

One of the many side effects of living without testosterone is loss of libido or sexual desire. This is something foreign to most men and is often difficult to deal with. Men describe feeling very distressed about this, and this lack of libido extends into many different aspects of their lives. Men report missing the sensation of sexual interest toward their partners, but they also feel like something is missing in their everyday lives. They don't notice an attractive woman crossing the street, or they don't think about sex at all where previously they thought about it during the day and anticipated seeing their partner later on. Only about 10% of men retain sexual interest while on this therapy.

Lack of libido can be difficult to understand. It's not like the man is ignoring his partner out of choice, but rather he never thinks about sex, has no sexual feelings and absolutely no sexual interest. Along with this lack of libido, the lack of testosterone also causes problems with erections. But most do not even notice that because sex doesn't even enter their minds anymore.

There really is no treatment for this lack of interest. Most men will no longer spontaneously touch their partner, so it may be up to the partner to do the touching. This can be challenging if the man used to initiate sexual activity. On the other hand, sometimes the partner is not upset by this lack of interest, and the two of them are happy to live in a nonsexual relationship.

> ## Take-Away Points
>
> - Try not to blame yourself for this lack of interest; it results from the medication and is not your fault.
> - If this causes stress with your partner, you may have to find ways to prompt yourself to give physical attention to your partner.
> - One way to do this is to remind yourself to touch or kiss your partner when the evening news starts, or when you get into bed. The impulse to do this may have vanished, but you can use prompts to remind yourself to act like the old you.
> - Your partner may have to initiate sexual touching even if this is not something he or she would usually do.

Talking It Out

Ted continued with the injections every three months. At his visits to the urologist, he mostly saw the nurse. His time with the urologist was very short, two to three minutes at the most, and it was difficult to ask any questions. The urologist was pleased with Ted's response to the androgen deprivation, which seemed to be all he wanted to mention at Ted's appointments before he left the room. Ted felt frustrated at these visits, but, as Joan pointed out, the nurse was very helpful.

After he had been on the injections for a year, he found the courage to ask the nurse about his lack of sexual interest. Joan had wanted him to ask about this long before, but he sometimes forgot when he was at the appointment, or else he felt stupid asking about this. The nurse seemed interested in his questions. She listened quietly as Ted described his lack of interest in sex and, of course, his inability to have an erection if he thought about it, which never happened anymore. "That's all perfectly normal for someone on androgen deprivation," she said. "Remember we talked about this when I first met you. Or maybe you don't remember at all. I know it's a lot to take in when you first hear about it."

The nurse seemed so comfortable with his recitation of everything that had gone wrong with his sex life that Ted was able to listen to her as she talked. She explained to him how the lack of testosterone was affecting his sex life. She encouraged him to ask questions and gave him information even without his having to ask. He already knew about lack of interest, but other effects were possible too. He was surprised to learn that over time, the amount of ejaculate his body produced would lessen until there was almost nothing. And he was disappointed to learn that the pills many of his friends took to help with erections would not help him. He didn't really care all that much about sex anymore, but what would Joan say?

Dr. Katz Explains

Not only do men lose interest in sex, but they also have no ejaculate because the lack of testosterone halts sperm production. Over time, the lack of testosterone also appears to change the structure of the muscles and elastic fibers in the penis itself. This results in something called venous leak; the chambers of the penis that usually fill with blood during an erection are not able to keep the blood trapped, and so erections cannot be maintained. This means that drugs such as Viagra® (Pfizer Inc.), Cialis® (Eli Lilly and Co.), and Levitra® (Bayer HealthCare Pharmaceuticals Inc.) will not work because all they do is prevent blood from leaving the spongy tissue of the penis. If the blood can't be trapped inside those tissues, the man will not be able to maintain an erection. Options for having an erection while on androgen deprivation include penile self-injection and penile implants. But for most men, their loss of interest in sex means that these options are not considered.

Body Wars

The months went by. Ted was tired often and for the first time in his life had started taking naps in the afternoon. They didn't really help all that much, but he didn't know what else to do. The hot flashes were still pretty bad, but he had learned to deal with them; he hardly ever wore a sweater inside the house and had given up on drinking hot liquids. He and Joan had spent long hours talking about how their sex life had changed; it had all but disappeared, and they both were very sad about that. He tried to remember to hug her, but the reality was that if she didn't initiate something, then he would just forget about it.

The other thing that greatly bothered him was how his body had changed. He had developed a ring of fat around his hips and had even grown breasts! All of this was really embarrassing. He hated wearing anything that clung to his body, and he had taken to wearing baggy clothes or sweaters when he went out, which caused problems with temperature control and hot flashes. He had tried working out more but to no effect. His skin felt very soft and he noticed that he had to shave less often. Joan sometimes joked that it was like living with his sister; he tried to smile, but that really hurt.

Dr. Katz Explains

Ted is experiencing many of the typical side effects of androgen deprivation. He has put on weight in the form of increased fat on his hips and abdomen. He has also developed breasts, a condition called gynecomastia. This can be somewhat painful, and some men have a short course of radiation treatment to the chest wall to alleviate this. Men also lose muscle mass and strength, and this combined with weight gain can be upsetting.

Take-Away Points

- Even if exercise doesn't seem to be helping with weight gain or loss of muscle strength, it is important to continue with it because of its benefits to your bones and heart.
- Eat healthily and do not smoke—poor diet and nicotine will only make matters worse.

One of the challenges of the weight gain and muscle loss is that increasing exercise doesn't really help. But regular exercise is especially important because the long-term use of androgen deprivation therapy has also been linked with the development of diabetes and bone loss. Other side effects of this treatment include difficulty concentrating and anemia. It is important to report any new signs or symptoms to your physician, and some recommend that men on androgen deprivation therapy have a bone scan at the beginning of treatment and every two years while on treatment.

Resignation and Hope

Eighteen months later, things were pretty much the same. Ted had gained almost 15 pounds despite exercising every day and cutting down on the amount of food he was eating. He was also much more forgetful, and occasionally this led to fights with Joan. He got really frustrated when she reminded him of something that he had forgotten, and he lashed out at her.

His PSA remained at a very low level, and his hip did not bother him at all. He had another bone scan about a year after he started the treatment, and there had been no progression, so he was happy about that. But every time he looked in the mirror he just wanted to close his eyes. He looked so different. Like the Michelin Man. Joan told him to get over himself, but he couldn't get over what he looked like. He looked like a giant marshmallow.

He talked to his family physician about it when he went for his annual checkup. Dr. Bryant was sympathetic and made some suggestions about diet and exercise, but Ted assured him that he was doing all of that. Dr. Bryant promised he would do some reading about the topic and suggested that Ted come back at the end of the month to review the results of the blood tests he had that day.

When he went back to see Dr. Bryant, Ted was pleased to learn that his cholesterol was under control and his PSA remained very low. Dr. Bryant then told him that he had read an article about androgen deprivation therapy that said some doctors prescribed intermittent therapy. What that meant was that some men did not stay on the androgen deprivation therapy permanently but went off it once their PSA was really low. They could stay off the medication, sometimes for many months, but as soon as their PSA started to rise, they had to go back on it. Ted felt his heart beat faster. Maybe this could work for him! Dr. Bryant promised to talk to the urologist about this, and Ted went home with hope in his heart for the first time in many months.

Dr. Katz Explains

Ted has now been on androgen depriva-tion therapy for well over a year. The cancer has responded to the lack of testosterone as measured by both the fall in PSA as well as the control of the bone cancer in his hip. Ted has been on continuous androgen deprivation therapy and is suffering many of the side effects. Another option is intermittent therapy, where the medication is stopped once the PSA has dropped to very low or undetectable levels and then the man stays off it until the PSA starts to rise again. Although we do not know if one method is better than the other, many urologists allow their patients to do this because they feel so much better during the time they are off the medication. Some urologists are comfortable with this approach, whereas others are not.

Take-Away Points

- Talk to your doctor about this approach to androgen deprivation. New findings are being published all the time, and the manage-ment of prostate cancer is changing.
- Engage your family doctor in your ongoing care; he or she knows you well and can be a useful ally in your treatment by providing you with information or advo-cating on your behalf with specialists.

Changes

The next time Ted went to see the urologist, he took Joan with him. She had not come to every appointment with him; they were so quick that there really didn't seem to be any point. This time she was with him, and she had a list of questions written out in her neat handwriting on a piece of paper.

The urologist mentioned that he'd had a call from Dr. Bryant. If Ted felt strongly about it, he was willing to stop the injections and see what happened. He explained the risks—the bone cancer might come back, his PSA could go up again—but he understood that it was difficult to be on the medication. Ted's relief was immense. Joan crumpled the piece of paper in her hand and smiled. They left the office that day hand in hand. And with hope.

CHAPTER 4

Erectile Dysfunction

I don't feel like a man anymore.

Erectile dysfunction is common after treatment for cancer and causes great distress to men and their partners. The ability to have an erection is something that for many men goes beyond what happens in the bedroom. Erections are symbolic of masculinity, and although no one else needs to know that a man can't have an erection, it is still something that causes great shame for many men when they encounter difficulties.

Loss of erections is also a very common side effect of the surgery commonly used to treat prostate cancer. Despite advances in surgical technique, it is very common for men to have great difficulty achieving erections after the surgery. This causes significant distress for the man and often affects his primary intimate relationship.

In this chapter, you will meet Brian, a 52-year-old man with prostate cancer. Despite his young age and successful surgery, Brian is not able to have erections one year after his surgery and is frustrated and angry.

From Brian's story, you will learn
- How erections are affected by surgery for prostate cancer
- What can be done to minimize the damage to erectile tissue
- How couples can work to find a different way of pleasing each other.

Brian's Story

Brian always expected he would get prostate cancer. He just saw it as his fate. His father had it in his 60s, and his older brother Steve was diagnosed two years ago at the age of 58. Because of his father's diagnosis, Brian's family doctor had advised him to have a yearly prostate-specific antigen (PSA) test and digital rectal exam starting in his 40s. He was not thrilled at the prospect but knew it made sense, so every year he went for a physical exam and blood test. The first few years he was really anxious; he didn't sleep well the week before and after the doctor's visit. But year after year, everything was fine. His doctor told him that his prostate felt like that of a 39-year-old, and every year his PSA test was within normal limits for a man his age.

The year he turned 50 was the first time that he wasn't nervous about the test results. He and his wife, Ginny, were going on a cruise to celebrate his 50th birthday, and he was really busy at work. He went to the lab, had his blood drawn, and rushed off to do some last-minute shopping. Later that week he saw his family doctor and was stunned to learn that there had been a small jump in his PSA, and the doctor was recommending a prostate biopsy. Why was this happening now?

Dr. Katz Explains

Although our knowledge of cancer genetics is far from complete, we are learning more and more about it every year. We know that when a man has a first-degree relative (a father or brother) with prostate cancer, his risk for developing this cancer is doubled. If he has two first-degree relatives, his risk is even higher. Men with a family history such as Brian's are advised to start PSA screening in their 40s or at least five years before the age at which their first-degree relative was diagnosed.

The PSA test is a screening test for prostate cancer. The use of this test is controversial because there is no evidence that the PSA test actually saves lives. Having the PSA test leads to a cascade of further testing, including a biopsy, which is invasive and carries the risk of bleeding and infection. And prostate cancer itself is not a very lethal cancer; the vast majority of men diagnosed with prostate cancer do not die of the disease. The treatments for prostate cancer cause significant challenges to quality of life, and many question whether it needs to be treated at all. However, many men do have this test, and many will say that having the test saved their life.

The Testing Begins

Brian was shocked and a bit confused by what his doctor was recommending. Why did this have to happen now? They were leaving that weekend for the cruise, and he had so much to do. He really didn't feel like dealing with all of this now, but at the same time, he did not want to go away with this hanging over his head. His doctor assured him that he could wait until after his vacation to have the biopsy, and it was unlikely that he would get an appointment with the urologist before then anyway. The doctor reassured Brian that his prostate felt fine with no obvious abnormalities and they were just being cautious.

He told Ginny about what had happened when he called her from the car as he was driving from the appointment. Ginny was the more rational of the two of them, and she calmed him down quickly. As a nurse, she had seen all sorts of things during her long career, and she had a wonderful ability to put everything in perspective. She calmly repeated most of what his family doctor had said, and within minutes Brian felt better and went back to work.

They left on the weekend for the long-awaited cruise. Brian even managed to not think about the test results until they boarded the plane for their flight home. The cruise had been wonderful, and the busy days and late nights had taken his mind off of what lay ahead. When they got home, there was a message from the doctor's office that he had an appointment with the urologist for the following Friday. He immediately felt anxious, but Ginny once again managed to calm him down. She told him she was going to the appointment with him, and there was nothing he could do to stop her. The relief was visible on his face and he reached out to hold her, more to comfort himself than anything else.

Friday came all too soon. Ginny picked him up at his office, and they drove together to the urologist's office, which was on the other side of town. The offices were very fancy—Ginny started to say something about the amount of money he must be making but then stopped herself. She could see that Brian was too anxious to appreciate her rather dry sense of humor. Fortunately, they did not have to wait long, and they were shown to a large examination room. Within five minutes a tall, thin man with a slight Irish accent entered the room after knocking quietly. Dr. Manley introduced himself and sat down at the computer in front of the desk in the corner of the room.

"Hmm . . ." he began in his soft, lilting voice. "I see your PSA went up a bit this last year. Not sure there's anything to worry about, but let's examine you and go from there." He looked up at Ginny from over his glasses. "You'd best wait out in the waiting room. I'll call you if there's anything you need to know." Ginny was somewhat surprised that she was being dismissed so early in the appointment, but she left the room without saying anything. She glanced at Brian's face as she moved toward the door, and it was white and pinched and he looked like he was about to cry.

Five minutes later Brian appeared in the waiting room. His face was still white but there were two spots of red on his cheeks. "Why did you just leave like that?" he hissed at Ginny. "Did I have a choice?" she whispered back. "He virtually threw me out the room!" Brian didn't answer her and instead went to the reception desk and waited while the young woman sitting there finished a phone conversation. She handed a slip of paper to Brian; he stuffed it into his jacket pocket and moved toward the door. Ginny had to hurry to catch up with him. He hardly spoke in the car, and Ginny knew better than to push him. Just as they drew up to his building he blurted it all out: "I have to have a biopsy. He felt something on my prostate. I just know it's cancer. I don't think I can do this!"

Dr. Katz Explains

A rise in PSA usually precipitates more invasive testing such as a biopsy. There is usually not a huge rush to have the biopsy, and the short delay while Brian and Ginny were on vacation was not going to change anything. The urologist had felt an abnormality on Brian's prostate although his family physician had not; this is not unusual. The digital rectal exam is a subjective test of what the healthcare provider feels; the fact that the urologist felt something but the family physician did not has more to do with who is doing the examination—their skill as well as how aggressive they are in examining the prostate.

The Walls Came Tumbling Down

The next week Brian had the biopsy. He was very nervous and did not sleep much in the days leading up to the test. He had to take antibiotics, which upset his stomach a little, and he was generally very stressed and unhappy. Ginny insisted on coming with him to the appointment even though she had to take off work to be there with him. He didn't say anything, but she could tell he was pleased to have her there.

Ginny was not allowed to accompany him when he had the actual procedure, but she sat with him in the examination room while he waited. They didn't talk much, and she held his hand until a nurse appeared and sent her out of the room. Twenty minutes later, the nurse came into the waiting room and said they were done and Brian was getting dressed. She said Brian would need to stay for about 15 minutes to make sure there was no bleeding. Soon after that, Brian entered the waiting room. He looked relieved that it was over but was a little shaky. Ginny asked if he'd had breakfast, and he sheepishly shook his head. She rummaged in her purse and found a granola bar, slightly dented but still whole and in its wrapper, and Brian took it from her and ate it quickly. At the 15-minute mark he went to the restroom to check if there was any bleeding, and to his relief there was none, and they could leave.

They went back to the same office a week later to hear the results of the biopsy. It had been a difficult week for him and Ginny. He had not slept well and was extremely anxious; he wouldn't or perhaps couldn't talk to Ginny about this, which made her feel helpless. As a nurse she was used to fixing things and people, and she was not used to this feeling of being unable to ease his anxiety.

The urologist entered the exam room where they were waiting and got right down to the point: "You have prostate cancer, I'm afraid. Low volume, low risk, but you need to get it out. I have a copy of the results for you, and you can take some time to think about what you want to do. My nurse will also give you some reading material and some Web sites that may be helpful. No big rush, but you need to do something. Any questions?"

Ginny and Brian felt the air leave the room. They were both stunned and could only shake their heads. The urologist shook their hands and then left the room as quickly as he had entered it. Ginny could not even look at Brian; she was afraid both to see his face and for him to see hers. Luckily, there was a knock on the door, and the nurse, the same one who had been there for the biopsy, entered the room. She had a large white envelope in her hands. She handed the envelope to Ginny, asked them if they had any additional questions, and gave them a card with a date and time for another appointment to see the urologist. Brian and Ginny were left in the room, speechless and stunned.

Take-Away Points

- Always take someone with you to an appointment where you will be receiving test results; you don't know what your reaction will be even if you are prepared for the worst.
- Make sure that you have an appointment to come back, preferably within a week, to discuss the results and ask questions.

Dr. Katz Explains

It is very common to be shocked when you hear the words "you have cancer," even if you were preparing for them or even expected them. Ginny and Brian's response is normal, and we know that people generally hear only 10% of the information that is given to them after those words. The urologist did not give them much time to think or react after he told them that Brian had prostate cancer; however, he also did not give them any additional information. There is both good and bad with this. The nurse gave them a package of information and also did not spend much time with them.

Quick Decisions

Ginny and Brian didn't talk much in the car on the way home. Later that evening Ginny asked Brian if she could read the information that the nurse had given them, and Brian snapped at her, "It's a free world, Ginny. Anyone can read that junk." Ginny stared at him and said, "I'm not the enemy here, Brian. We're together in this. We have to be." Brian's face crumpled as the words came out of her mouth. "I know, Gin," he mumbled. "I'm sorry. I'm just so damn scared."

Ginny wrapped her arms around him. "I know you're scared. I am too. But we're in this together, and maybe not today, but soon, you have to read all that stuff and make a decision about what you're going to do." Brian nodded his head and folded his arms around her. She was right. He had to decide.

Later that day he talked to his brother, who had surgery as his treatment two years ago. His brother was emphatic in his advice to Brian. "Just have the surgery!" he said. "Just get it out and then it's done." Brian and his brother had never been close, and he was reluctant to ask him any more questions. "This is really bad luck," said his brother. "First the old man, then me, and now you. Runs in the genes, I guess." Their call ended with Brian wondering why his brother was not more sympathetic, but that was history and he had to move forward now.

That evening he opened the package of information the nurse had given him. Inside were a number of glossy brochures, and when he paged through them, they all seemed to say the same thing: the choice of treatment is a personal one, talk to your doctor, things will be okay. Ginny had read the information earlier that day, and even though she was a nurse, she was confused by the lack of clear direction in all of the pamphlets.

"I've made up my mind," Brian announced. "I'm going to have the surgery. I don't want to talk about it. I just want to do it." Ginny knew that voice; once he made up his mind about something, he would not budge. She was the more questioning one, she would have talked to people, researched things on the Internet, but that was not how Brian did things. At least he had made up his mind and now they could make plans and move forward.

Dr. Katz Explains

Making a decision about what treatment to have for prostate cancer is difficult. Surgery and radiation have the same success rates in terms of curing the cancer. But each kind of treatment carries with it a significant burden of side effects. These side effects influence quality of life, and only the man himself can decide what those side effects would mean in his life. The major side effects after surgery are incontinence (inability to control the bladder) and erectile difficulties. These may improve over time; however, there is no guarantee of that. After radiation, a man can expect a frequent urge to urinate and pain on urination, as well as some rectal irritation leading to diarrhea and pain. These usually resolve over time but may persist in the long term. Erectile difficulties usually occur one to two years after completion of radiation treatment.

Take-Away Points

- Take your time when making a treatment decision.
- Consider all the options and read as much as you can.
- Be careful when talking to other men who have been treated for prostate cancer; you do not know the details about their cancer, and it may be at a very different stage than yours.
- Only you can decide what side effects you are prepared to live with.

It is important to take as much time as you need to make the decision about what kind of treatment you will have; in most instances today, the cancer is diagnosed at an early stage, and because prostate cancer tends to be slow growing, there is usually time to make the decision about treatment with no rush. However, some men may be diagnosed when the cancer is more aggressive or advanced, and they may not have any choice in the kind of treatment they will have.

A Man on a Mission

Once Brian had made up his mind, he was a man on a mission. He called the urologist's office and insisted on seeing the doctor the next day. Within a week he had completed all the blood tests and other investigations he needed prior to surgery. Exactly two weeks after he received the diagnosis, Brian was under anesthetic, having the surgery. He stayed in the hospital for two days, and most of the time he slept. He was eager to get home and persuaded the doctor to let him leave early because Ginny was a nurse. The first few days at home were difficult for him; he had an indwelling catheter that irritated him, and he was grumpy most of the time. Ginny just kept her mouth shut and didn't argue with him. Once the first week had passed, his mood improved, and he was really happy the day the catheter came out.

The days went slowly for him during the recovery period. He had been instructed to take six weeks off work, and after the first three, he was really bored. He always thought that it would be nice to stay home all day and watch television, but he discovered that daytime television was not all that great. He had never been much of a reader, so he did not touch any of the books that Ginny had taken out the library for him. The hours went by slowly, and by the fourth week he was ready to go back to work. He talked to his boss, and they agreed that he could come back for a couple of hours a day initially and slowly build up to regular hours. His work was not all that strenuous, but it did require him to be on his feet a lot. The first few days were exhausting, and he wondered if he had made the right decision to go back so early.

The Six-Week Checkup

Once again Brian found himself in the urologist's waiting room with a racing heart and sweaty palms. Ginny was with him, and they sat in silence, waiting to be called to hear the important news about the pathology results from the surgery. It was 30 minutes before they were called, and then they waited another 20 minutes before the urologist entered the examination room where they were waiting.

"'Morning, Brian," the urologist said as he entered the room. In his hand were some papers, and he read them quickly as he sat down. "Everything looks really good from the surgery. The pathology report says that we got it all, and you should be in the clear. How are you doing with the bladder control? Good?" Brian did not answer immediately. He was still trying to process the information about the pathology, and he did not quite know how to answer the question about his bladder. He was having a lot of leakage at work and hated that he had to wear a diaper, but he couldn't risk having an accident in front of all the guys on the line.

"My nurse will be in shortly to talk to you about getting erections back," the doctor continued. "Shouldn't be a problem because I spared the nerves, but she has a lot of information for you." Once again the urologist shook their hands and was gone. Ginny and Brian looked at each other; could it be that their luck had changed? It sounded like everything was okay, but they didn't have much time to talk to him.

A few minutes later, the nurse came into the room. She once again had a package of information in her hand. "Let's get you started on our penile rehab program, Brian," she said as she sat down. "I'm sure you read about it in the last package I gave you, but here's some more information to remind you. You're going to be taking a small dose of Viagra (also known as sildenafil) every night before you go to bed. If you don't see the return of erections soon after that, we're going to need to talk about other strategies. Here's a prescription that you should fill today, and start taking the pills tonight. Any questions?" Once again Ginny and Brian shook their heads. They did have questions, many questions, but everything felt so rushed. Brian felt stupid that he couldn't remember anything about this from the other package of reading material. The past weeks had been such a blur, and now he had something else to worry about. When was it going to end?

Dr. Katz Explains

It is quite common today for men to be encouraged to take medication following surgery to maximize the chances that erections return; this is known as penile rehabilitation. Even with nerve-sparing surgery, the nerves go into shock after being manipulated during the surgery. This not only results in an inability to have an erection for sexual purposes, but it also causes the man to no longer have the three to six erections he has while asleep. The purpose of these nonsexual erections seems to be to keep the tissues of the penis well nourished and well oxygenated. Without these regular erections, the tissues of the penis undergo changes that make the return of normal erections almost impossible and also affect the ability of the penis to respond to medications such as Viagra (sildenafil), Cialis (tadalafil), or Levitra (vardenafil).

One approach of penile rehabilitation is for the man to ensure that he has an erection two to three times a week; this can involve self- or partner stimulation. If the man is not having erections in response to genital stimulation, then he should start using penile self-injection two to three times a week to ensure that blood is getting into the penis. Another approach is for the man to take a low nightly dose of either Viagra or Levitra (Cialis lasts about 36 hours in the bloodstream, so this particular medication may be taken every second night). While on this regimen, it is recommended that men try to achieve regular erections at least twice a week.

Not all urologists incorporate penile rehabilitation in their practice, but it is important to ask what can be done about encouraging the return of erections because if more four months go by without regular erections, the damage to penile tissues may be so bad that spontaneous erections will never return.

The Months Go By

Things went back to normal quite quickly after that. Brian was back at work full time, and within three months he no longer had any urine leakage and eventually stopped wearing the diapers. He probably wore them for a number of weeks longer than he should have, but he was so scared of having an accident. His energy level was soon back to normal, and except for the scar on his abdomen, he felt like the old Brian. The months flew by, and soon it was the first anniversary of his surgery.

There was one area where things were not back to normal. It had been almost 12 months since he had an erection. This bothered him more than he liked to admit. He joked about it to Ginny, and she responded as if it was really a joke, but she could tell that he was bothered, and she didn't know what to say.

He had been taking Viagra every night, but there had been little response. He had read the material the nurse gave him those many months ago, but the thought of injecting himself in the penis was too much. He did notice that when he washed himself in the shower there appeared to be some thickening of his penis in response to his touch, but that was all there was. The other thing that really bothered him was the fact that his penis had shrunk. Sometimes it seemed to have gone right up into his stomach, like it did if he swam in the cold ocean. Ginny had noticed that he always wore pajamas to bed, whereas before he didn't. She asked him about it once and he told her he was feeling cold, and she never asked again.

He had gone back to see the urologist every three months, and the topic of erections never came up. The nurse waved at him from behind the reception desk, but he never talked to her again. The urologist provided him with another prescription for Viagra and he kept taking the medication every night, but it did not seem to be working. A year after his surgery, he went to see his family physician for his annual physical. Dr. Cummings was about the same age as Brian and very thorough. He asked him about his recovery from the surgery and seemed surprised when Brian admitted that he could not have an erection. "That seems strange to me," he said. "I'm going to send you to a colleague of mine who has a special interest in this. She may have something to offer that could help."

Take-Away Points

- Using medications like Viagra, Cialis, and Levitra regularly may prevent shrinkage of the penis, but we do not have strong evidence that this is useful yet.
- Getting blood and therefore oxygen and other nutrients into the penis regularly may also help to prevent shrinkage, so self- or partner stimulation is important.
- Some men find that using a vacuum pump three times a week helps to draw blood into the penis and prevents penile shrinkage.

Dr. Katz Explains

It can take as long as 18–24 months for erectile functioning to return, and many men get frustrated with the lack of erections way before that. It is important to have realistic expectations about the length of time this may take. Many men also assume that the medications advertised for erectile dysfunction will work for them; the fact is that they may help 50% of men, depending on the degree of nerve sparing that was performed. Men find that they have to consider something more invasive or mechanical such as a vacuum pump, intraurethral pellet (alprostadil, MUSE®, Vivus, Inc.), or penile self-injection.

Penile shortening is also very common after radical prostatectomy, and many patients are not warned about this. It often comes as a shock when the man looks at himself naked in the mirror! In the first six months after surgery, the penis often looks as though it has shrunk inside the body. This happens because while the erection nerves are recovering, other nerves are more active, and it is these nerves that pull the penis backward into the abdomen, much like what happens when a man enters cold water. If you grab the end of the penis and stretch it gently, it will stretch to its full length. The contraction nerves will become less dominant as the other nerves recover over time, so this type of shortening is usually temporary if nerve-sparing surgery was performed.

The second reason for penile shrinkage tends to occur over the long term because of the lack of oxygen and nutrients reaching the penile tissue. The tissue shrinks because of lack of nutrition, and these changes tend to be permanent. People often think that the penis shrinks because a piece of the urethra has been removed when the prostate gland was removed. This is not the cause of the shrinkage because the remaining urethra and bladder are pulled down and anchored to the muscles of the pelvic floor and cannot be pulled backward into the body.

The Sex Therapist

Brian was a bit surprised when a week later he received a call from a woman who introduced herself over the phone as the sex therapist who had received a referral from Dr. Cummings, his family physician. Her voice was warm and friendly, and she asked Brian if he would like to come in with his partner to see her to discuss what was happening. He agreed, and they made an appointment for the end of the week.

Ginny was a little surprised that Brian had made the appointment without talking to her first, but she was keen to see him get some help. Over the past few months they had really drifted apart. Brian hardly ever kissed her anymore, and he tensed up when she tried to touch him, so she just stopped. If this therapist could help, then she was willing to go along.

The afternoon of the appointment, Brian seemed really on edge. Ginny tried to joke about it, but he just snapped at her, so she spent the rest of the ride in silence with a lump in her throat from trying not to cry. The therapist opened the door to her office within seconds of their knock. She was about their age, in her 50s, and was short with curly brown hair. Her brown eyes were warm and her smile wide and genuine. "Come on in, please, and make yourselves comfortable," she said. The room was filled with soft light from three wall sconces, and there was a grouping of leather furniture in the middle of the room. Ginny and Brian sat on a worn but comfortable sofa, and the specialist sat opposite them in a big armchair.

"Let's begin," Brian said, surprised to hear the words tumble out of his mouth. It was as if he had suddenly found the words to express all his feelings from the past year. He talked without stopping for 20 minutes about his frustration and loss and fears. Ginny sat in stunned silence; she had suspected only a fraction of his pain. The two women listened as Brian talked about no longer feeling like a man and his fears that Ginny would leave him to find someone who could satisfy her sexually. She started to interrupt him, but the therapist held up her hand to stop her. Only when Brian finally stopped talking did she ask Ginny to voice her thoughts.

Ginny barely knew where to begin. With tears in her eyes, she pleaded with him to hear that she would not leave him because he could not have an erection. In an attempt at humor she said that his thinking these thoughts were grounds for her leaving, but for another man, never. Brian did not make eye contact with her as she described her feelings of loneliness in the year since his surgery. She talked hesitantly about how isolated she felt and how she missed the touching that was a big part of their lives. As she talked, Brian reached out and took her hand. She looked down at where their hands were joined, and tears flooded her eyes.

Dr. Katz Explains

It is interesting how it can be so difficult to talk to your partner about something like sex. Some people are able to talk openly and honestly about it while other couples struggle. Brian and Ginny are an example of a couple for whom not talking about the problem has led to misunderstandings and assumptions that are causing a great deal of distress. Talking to each other with an objective and skilled professional present can be really helpful. The therapist (or social worker, psychologist, or counselor) provides a degree of safety that things will not get out of control and can help both partners to express themselves without interruption and can also maintain a nonthreatening environment.

Brian and Ginny are expressing feelings that are very common when a couple's usual sex life is threatened: She feels lonely because touching has stopped, and he feels like he is no longer a man. He may stop touching her in the belief that touching must lead to intercourse and that it is leading her on because he cannot perform.

Finding Solutions

The therapist asked many questions after Ginny and Brian stopped talking. She asked them about the meaning of intercourse in their lives and what, if anything, they had done to accommodate the change after Brian's surgery. She also asked about what Brian had tried to help him have erections and if anything had worked. Brian responded that the pills did not seem to be working, and he was frustrated because all the ads he had seen made it appear that this was something easily treated. Ginny reminded him that the ads were perhaps overly optimistic and not aimed at men who had surgery for prostate cancer. The therapist smiled; this couple were doing and saying the right things!

The therapist asked Brian if he had experienced an orgasm since his surgery, and he looked at her in disbelief. How could that happen if he wasn't having erections? She also asked Ginny about her preferred sexual activities, and Ginny admitted that the only way she could have an orgasm was with oral or manual stimulation and that intercourse itself was far less important to her. Brian reacted as if this were the first time he had ever heard of this. And so the therapist made some suggestions, and both Brian and Ginny suddenly saw some hope.

Dr. Katz Explains

This may be the first time that this couple has actually talked about their preferences regarding sexual activity. Strange as it may seem, many couples never talk about this and just go along with what their partner seems to like, want, and do. No one had told Brian that he could still experience an orgasm even without an erection. Many men assume that an erection is an essential part of sexual satisfaction because their experience has been one of a series of steps: erection, penetration, orgasm. Orgasms are caused by a spinal cord reflex that is not affected by the surgery to remove the prostate. With stimulation of the penis and scrotum, most men will have an orgasm even though the penis is flaccid. Ginny has also disclosed that, like many women, she achieves an orgasm not through penetration but with oral and manual stimulation. Perhaps this may be enough for this couple, who may be able to alter their usual pattern of sexual activity and focus on mutual masturbation and/or oral-genital stimulation and place less emphasis on penetration.

Take-Away Points

- It takes some effort to even think about doing things differently in the face of sexual changes after treatment, but it can be very helpful to find out that both you and your partner can achieve satisfaction through other means.
- Many couples find great enjoyment in doing things differently, but some find it difficult to maintain new practices and just want things to be the way they were.
- Find out who in your community has a practice in sex therapy, sexuality counseling, or sexual medicine. A referral to a professional can be of great benefit.

A New Journey

Brian and Ginny left their appointment with the therapist feeling drained but also hopeful. They had talked to each other in a way that they had probably never done in the past. They had a deeper understanding of each other's feelings, and Ginny especially was hopeful that they had opened the door to better communication about something that was both important yet scary to talk about. That night she took special care as she made dinner and even opened a bottle of their favorite wine. Maybe tonight . . .

CHAPTER 5

Pain With Orgasm

It feels like a kick in the groin, and that's not good.

Many men experience changes to their orgasms following pelvic or bowel surgery. They may experience many different altered sensations, including difficulty reaching orgasm. In this chapter, you will read about Steve, who had a family history of colon cancer and was diagnosed himself three years ago. He had extensive surgery to remove all of his large intestine. He is able to have erections, but his orgasms are painful, and this has led him to avoid sexual activity because of fear of the pain.

Pain with orgasm is not normal and can come as a shock to a man when something usually associated with great pleasure suddenly is painful. Some men cope with this by avoiding sexual activity; this results in changes to their primary relationship and affects the man's quality of life. Other men talk about this to their healthcare provider and seek assistance to solve this problem.

At the end of this chapter, you will learn about

• The effects of major abdominal surgery on the pelvic floor muscles
• How to seek help for this condition
• How pelvic floor physiotherapy can offer relief from this condition.

Steve's Story

Steve, who is 38 years old, has a strong family history of colon cancer with almost all of his uncles and aunts on his mother's side having been diagnosed with this cancer. Because of this, he was advised to have regular monitoring of his colon, and since he was a young man, he has complied. In his early twenties, he really hated it. He tried once or twice to skip his regular colonoscopy, but his mother asked him if he'd gone that year, and he couldn't lie to her. As he grew older he realized the importance of regular screening and just accepted it. He met Nancy the year he turned 28 and knew she was the one. It took a little persuading, but she eventually agreed to go out with him, and within six months they were engaged.

Nancy took over his mother's role as the one who reminded Steve to have his yearly examinations. They were thinking about starting a family, and it was more important than ever to him to take care of himself. They soon had a little girl named Amy, and she was followed two years later by baby Liam. Steve felt that his life was blessed; he had a perfect family and a pretty great life.

Four years ago he had a colonoscopy in March, his birth month, and when he woke up from the sedation, the gastrointestinal specialist had bad news for him. He had seen three polyps in his colon, which were removed for further inspection by the pathologist. The pathologist examined them and found that two were malignant. Steve and Nancy were devastated: He had always feared this legacy that appeared to dog his mother's family, and his greatest fear had come true. It was very difficult telling his mother the news. She was the only one in her family who had not been diagnosed with colon cancer, and she really hoped the streak had ended. She questioned why this should happen to her son when she was cancer-free, but of course there is no answer to this kind of question.

Steve was offered a choice of surgery: The surgeon could remove the part of the colon where the polyps were, but then Steve would need to continue with his yearly screenings and might need a colostomy bag to collect waste while the colon was healing. Or, the surgeon could remove the entire colon, effectively eliminating his risk of any polyps or cancer in the future. The second option was a much bigger surgery. It involved the creation of a pouch from the end of the small intestine that attached to the anus, allowing Steve to eliminate waste normally but with the risk that he could have multiple loose bowel movements each day. Neither option sounded great to him, but he eventually decided to have his entire colon removed. It just made more sense to him: get rid of the source of the problem and get on with life.

Steve had the surgery a month later. He knew it was major surgery, but he was not prepared for how bad he would feel after it. He had an ileostomy for the first couple of months. This meant that all his waste went into a bag attached to the front of his abdomen. He knew he would have this after the surgery, but he didn't know that it would bother him so much. His mother told him that he was actually lucky; he didn't need to have any other treatment for the cancer, and that was a very good thing. She described how his aunts and uncles had to endure chemotherapy or radiation after their surgery. But Steve didn't really listen; his suffering was overwhelming to him, and he just wanted to be left alone. He developed an infection somewhere inside him and was on antibiotics for weeks. The surgeon was concerned that he was not getting better, so one month after the first surgery they had to have a look inside him, where they found a large abscess that needed to be drained. He was in the hospital for a week after that surgery, and he lost even more weight and was as weak as a kitten.

Nancy and the kids got him through the months of recovery. Amy was now seven, and Liam was five. They were energetic children and asked lots of questions about everything, including the bag attached to Steve's abdomen. Amy wanted to touch it every chance she got. She seemed fascinated by the contents that sloshed around. Steve was horrified when she tried to look at it or touch it. Nancy suggested in her quiet way that if he had one-tenth of his daughter's acceptance, things would be much easier for him. He knew she was right but he couldn't help the way he felt.

Eventually the ileostomy was closed and he began to feel better. His weight was still down almost 15 pounds, and while Nancy teased him about being as sexy as he was when she met him, he didn't think that was amusing. He really didn't think that his recovery would be so long and complicated, but it was done now, and he looked forward to going back to work. It had been almost four months since he had cleaned up his desk at the law firm, and he hadn't had much contact with anyone there except for receiving some flowers while in the hospital and a fruit basket when he was discharged. He didn't want anyone to see him with the bag, and he was still reluctant to be seen looking so thin and weak.

Exactly four and a half months after his surgery he went back to work. He was nervous about this, but he knew it was time, and Nancy was pushing him hard to get back to normal life. He was having some difficulties adjusting to the loose bowel movements he had about five times a day and was worried that this would be embarrassing at work. He tried to avoid the foods that made it worse—mushrooms were a real problem—and made sure to go to the restroom every three hours to avoid an accident or the urgent need to empty his bowels while he was with a client. But he went back, and he managed.

Finding Each Other

Steve actually enjoyed being back at work. He was anxious about the lack of clients in his practice for the first two weeks, but soon his days filled up as his partners referred clients to him and some of his old clients came back. Every day he gained more strength and felt less exhausted at the day's end. Nancy could really see a change in him; he was more fun to be around and was more interested in playing with their children. Their 10th anniversary was approaching, and she wanted to do something special to mark the occasion as well as his recovery.

She made arrangements for them to spend the weekend in Minneapolis, which was a two-hour car ride from their house. She bought tickets to watch the Twins on Saturday afternoon. She made a reservation for dinner that night at the same restaurant they went to after he proposed. Steve's mother agreed to look after the children, and Nancy arranged with Steve's secretary to clear his calendar for Friday—and to keep it a secret. The night before, she packed a bag for him, and when he kissed her goodbye that morning as he prepared to leave for work, she surprised him with the news that he wasn't going to work but instead was heading out for a special weekend.

Steve was certainly surprised. In fact, he was shocked. For the first hour or so after the kids left for school, he wandered around the house, not really sure what he should do. Nancy had it all organized, however, and at 11 am they packed the car and left. As the miles flew past, his mood grew even lighter, and by the time they reached the outskirts of the city, he was smiling. Nancy even caught him whistling quietly.

They checked into the hotel, and Nancy threw herself onto the bed, landing on her back with her arms and legs spread, like a kid making a snow angel. Steve lay down next to her and suddenly they were kissing like giddy teenagers. The intensity of their feelings was overwhelming, and soon they were making love. It had been so long—five months—that it was soon over. As Steve reached orgasm, he cried out loudly. Nancy thought it was from pleasure, but there was something in the sound of his cry that made her open her eyes and look at his face. He was in pain! He fell onto the bed and immediately curled up into the fetal position. For a few minutes he lay there, his eyes closed, his knees drawn up to his chest.

Nancy's mind was racing. What could this be? After a while he opened his eyes and uncurled his body. "That was weird," he said. "I have never felt anything like that before. That really hurt." Nancy put her arms around him, and they talked about what had happened. Steve described a sharp and then throbbing pain deep in his pelvis that started just as he reached orgasm. "It feels like something's broken in there," he said softly. "How much more am I supposed to go through?" They lay in bed for a few hours. Nancy dozed off and on, and Steve must have as well because it was soon dusk and the light in the room changed.

They got up, showered, and went for dinner. Nancy could tell that Steve was trying his best to appear upbeat and as if he was enjoying himself. She asked him once or twice if he was okay. He nodded his head, but she could tell that he wasn't. When they got back to the hotel, he told her that he still had a deep ache in his pelvis, but it was bearable. The rest of the weekend was fun, but the memory of the incident colored their time away, and on Sunday they left early for the drive home.

Nancy assumed that Steve would contact his doctor to talk about what had happened. Their lives were so busy that it was two weeks before they had a chance to spend some time alone, and she asked what the doctor had said. Steve admitted that he hadn't talked to anyone about it. Nancy was speechless. They were both young, and sex was an important part of their lives before his surgery. Were they just not going to have sex again, ever? Steve was defensive as she pushed him to make an appointment; this was his problem and he would fix it. As if to prove her wrong, that night they made love, and the same thing happened. It was not as bad as before, and the throbbing went away after about 30 minutes, but the next morning Steve called his doctor.

Dr. Katz Explains

The pain that Steve experienced with orgasm is likely caused by scar tissue that has formed inside his abdomen and pelvis after the surgery he had to remove his colon. Additional scar tissue also developed as a result of the abscess that formed after the surgery and had to be drained. Some of this scar tissue may have attached itself to the muscles of the pelvic floor that lie in a sling from front to back under the bladder. The urethra and rectum pass through these muscles. During orgasm, these muscles contract rapidly, and anything that affects them will cause pain during orgasm.

This kind of internal damage is common after colon surgery. The muscles of the pelvic floor may become tight and stay contracted for long periods of time. This in itself can cause chronic pain or lead to problems with constipation. Because Steve only had this pain with orgasm, it is likely that this is an acute problem, but it can lead to more chronic problems and pain.

Seeking Help

Steve called the surgeon's office early the next morning. The receptionist explained that he was really booked up, but Steve insisted that he needed to be seen, even if he had to wait in the office waiting room until the doctor had a moment. The receptionist looked through his bookings and asked Steve if he could come in at the end of day with the understanding that it might be quite late before he was seen. Steve agreed and arrived at the doctor's office at 4:30 pm.

He waited for about 45 minutes and then was ushered into an examination room. Dr. Strong looked tired. Steve knew that he saw his hospital patients between 6 and 7 am and then had a full day in the office. The physician sat down on the small stool next to the desk and asked Steve why he was there. Steve was surprised at how difficult it was to say the words. He stammered and stuttered a bit, and the doctor sat patiently, waiting for him to describe his problem. Eventually Steve got the words out: "I had this pain, really bad, during sex. Umm, not all the time, just at the end, umm, during orgasm, you know?" His face was red and his hands were clenched in his lap. "I see," said Dr. Strong in a matter-of-fact voice. "This is something that we see quite commonly after the kind of surgery you've had." Steve was shocked. It was common! So why had nobody warned him?

Dr. Strong asked Steve to drop his pants and lie down on the examining table. Steve did as he was instructed to, but his mind was whirling with this new information. This happened often, and yet no one had told him! That was just not right. He felt Dr. Strong insert a gloved finger into his rectum, and Steve gasped with pain, "Ouch! Darn, that hurt!" Dr. Strong withdrew his finger, removed the glove, and patted Steve on the hip. "Just as I thought," he said. "You've got a lot of scar tissue in there. You're going to need some physiotherapy."

Dr. Katz Explains

It can be difficult to talk about sexual difficulties with healthcare providers for a variety of reasons. Most of us are not used to saying the words out loud to someone who is not an intimate partner. We often joke about sex, but talking about it seriously is much more difficult. Many healthcare providers do not ask questions about sex or sexual functioning as part of the routine care they provide. There are all sorts of reasons for this, and some may be good reasons, but not asking about it indicates to the patient that it is not important or not something that the doctor or nurse wants to talk about. Research shows that healthcare providers will talk about it if the patient asks, but the patient usually waits for the healthcare provider to ask! The result is a deafening silence with no questions asked and no answers given.

Take-Away Points

- If you have a question, ask it and don't stop asking until you get a satisfactory answer.
- Healthcare providers are willing to talk about the most sensitive topics, but you may have to ask first.

When Steve did ask about this, he was shocked to hear that the pain he was having was relatively common among people who have had colon surgery. He was justifiably annoyed that he was not told about the possibility of this before his surgery or at any other time. It is often difficult to tell patients everything that can possibly happen after treatment. Patients may experience information overload and not remember much at all. So, healthcare providers instinctively tell patients the most important things and then hopefully keep giving appropriate information over time. This latter part is where things often get forgotten.

A Different Sort of Massage

Steve received a call from the physiotherapist's office later that week. Dr. Strong had told him he was going to send the referral, but the response was really fast.

They set up an appointment for the next week. The receptionist told Steve that he would be seeing someone named Kelli and gave him directions to the clinic.

The appointment date arrived soon. Steve was a bit nervous—what was a pelvic floor physiotherapist anyway? He thought about asking Nancy to go with him but decided that he needed to deal with his problem on his own. Things had been a little tense between them recently. He was reluctant to have sex because he was afraid it would hurt, and Nancy seemed distant with him. Sex had always been important to them, and since his surgery it was as if they had lost a connection between each other. The first few months after the surgery he hadn't really noticed or missed sex, but he was feeling normal again, and now he missed it. But it hurt. It just seemed unfair.

The physiotherapist came into the waiting room to greet him. She introduced herself, and Steve sensed genuine warmth from her. They went into an office that was decorated with images of forests, and Kelli asked him to tell his story. He hardly knew where to start. He talked about the years of screening for cancer and the relief he felt when he had to make a decision about surgery. He described the pain and frustration with the recovery that went on for months. And then he talked about how at last he felt normal, and yet he still wasn't normal. With gentle prodding from the physiotherapist, Steve described the pain he felt during orgasm. He was a bit embarrassed when he told her that it had only happened twice because they had only had sex twice since his surgery. Kelli smiled and made a joke about how sex never happened as frequently as one's neighbors, and Steve felt himself relax.

Kelli then explained that she would need to do a rectal examination to learn more about what was happening. Steve visibly tensed up; the last time he had one of those it hurt a lot. Kelli smiled and said that he may be surprised at how different this examination would be. And she was right. She was gentle and told him exactly what she was going to do before she did it. She reminded him to breathe deeply, and before he knew it, the examination was over.

Kelli left the room so that Steve could get dressed. A few minutes later she escorted him to her office, a tranquil space with comfortable furniture and colorful art on the walls. She had a large set of diagrams on her desk and she began by explaining to him the structure and function of the pelvic floor muscles. Steve was not really interested in all of this; he wanted help and he wanted help fast. Kelli sensed his impatience and told him that this background information was essential to his future treatment. Steve tried hard to focus on what she was saying but after another five minutes blurted out his frustration. "Can you not just fix this? I am so tired of having to compromise and get used to life being different!"

Kelli took a deep breath; perhaps this patient really was different, and she agreed to get on with the treatment and leave the explanations for later. She explained to Steve that his treatment would consist of some exercises that he could do on his own as well as some massage of the pelvic floor muscles that she would do. Steve was curious: How was she going to massage his muscles? As he thought this, he realized what she meant. This was internal massage! Kelli just smiled as she saw his facial expression. "Yes, Steve. That's exactly what I'm going to do. You'll get used to it in time." Steve was not sure of that, but he agreed to start that day.

Once again he undressed and lay on the examination table. He covered himself with a sheet and waited for Kelli to come back. He was embarrassed and tense and was really glad that he had not told Nancy about this appointment. Kelli entered the room and in her gentle fashion explained what she was going to do. The cause of his pain was a combination of scar tissue buildup from the two surgeries as well as the muscles of the pelvic floor being too tense. The massage that she was going to do would relax the muscles as well as provide some stretching of the scar tissue. Steve just switched off his mind and let her do her work.

Dr. Katz Explains

A pelvic floor physiotherapist is a specialized professional who is an expert on the functioning of the pelvic floor muscles. Most people just ignore these important muscles, which support our internal organs and are an essential part of the process to eliminate waste. They also contract with orgasm, and this is why Steve had pain with orgasm. At an initial meeting with a pelvic floor physiotherapist, an assessment will be done and a treatment plan identified. Learning about how these muscles function is an important part of treatment, but as we have seen, Steve was not interested in this part of the plan!

For someone like Steve who has a large amount of internal scarring, massage of the scar tissue can be very helpful. In addition, the muscles of the pelvic floor

Take-Away Points

- Highly specialized health-care professionals are available in some centers to help with problems such as that which Steve is experiencing.
- Contact your state's physiotherapy board to find out about specialized physiotherapists in or near your hometown.

are often in a state of tension and do not relax properly. Gentle stretching of these muscles will help to normalize their tone and decrease pain. Steve will also need to do some relaxation exercises on his own to help with this.

Slow but Steady Wins the Race

Steve went to the physiotherapist three times a week. He still had not told Nancy about this; it felt weird that this attractive young woman was sticking her finger up his backside, and he wasn't sure what Nancy's reaction would be. As the weeks went by, he felt better physically, but he also realized that by not telling Nancy in the beginning, she was going to be even angrier if he told her now. He really was feeling much better. Kelli had given him some advice about diet and fluid intake. He usually ate only when he was hungry and ate whatever was on hand; sometimes that was cookies or pretzels at the office. His fluid intake was also poor; as a young lawyer he had limited his fluid intake to avoid needing to urinate while in court, and this habit had persisted even though he spent little time in court now. Kelli had explained the need for fiber and lots of water to prevent constipation, which would exacerbate his tense muscles. He found that with these changes in his diet he had much more regular bowel movements and very little diarrhea, something that had bothered him since his surgery.

Dr. Katz Explains

Taking care of one's body often involves changes that apply to more than one area of one's body or life. Steve found that his treatment with Kelli spilled over into his diet, and this in many ways seemed to make a bigger difference than just the massage.

Let's Try This One More Time

The weeks went by, and Steve found himself feeling so much better. Nancy had noticed that his mood had improved. He was less irritable and seemed more relaxed. She wanted to ask why but stopped herself. He almost seemed like his old self, and she was grateful for this. They still had not made love, and it had been almost three months now. She tried not to show how frustrated she was with this, but her patience was wearing thin. She made up her mind to talk to him after dinner that night.

She sent the kids to her parents and prepared a nice dinner for the two of them. Steve had been eating more salad recently, so she made a big bowl of greens with all sorts of interesting ingredients and a lovely homemade dressing. She even lit some candles and opened a bottle of their favorite wine. Steve seemed surprised to see how much effort she had gone to; he wondered if he had forgotten a special anniversary or birthday! They ate dinner quietly. Nancy told Steve about the kids' progress at school and in sports. Steve listened and then talked a bit about what was happening in his law firm. Neither of them wanted to get up from the table after they finished eating. There seemed to be something unspoken in the air between them. They both started talking at once. Steve wanted to confess about the physiotherapist, and Nancy wanted to talk about getting some help for their nonexistent sex life.

As the words poured out of both of them, they stopped to listen. Steve told Nancy about going to the physiotherapist and how much better he was feeling. Nancy told him how frustrated she was by the lack of intimacy in their life. After these disclosures, they sat in silence for a few moments. They had kept so much from each other.

Nancy glanced at her watch; the kids didn't need to be picked up for another hour or more. Could they try one more time? Steve seemed hesitant—he was afraid that sex would hurt. But part of him knew that he had to try. Kelli had talked about this at their last appointment, and he knew that he had to find out if there had been improvement. For the first time in their entire relationship, Steve felt shy. Nancy sensed this and took his hand, leading him gently to their bedroom, where two children had been conceived and where the couple had spent many hours sharing their love.

To both of their delight, things were fine. Steve had no pain. "It's kind of like riding a bicycle, I guess," he murmured as he fell asleep, his arms wrapped around his wife. "I thought I'd forgotten how to do it!"

CHAPTER 6

Altered Body Image

How could anyone love me with the way I look?

This chapter covers body image, which is one of the most significant changes and influences on sexuality and is almost universally experienced as part of the cancer trajectory. Bob is 67 years old and has bladder cancer. He now passes urine into a bag on the outside of his abdomen. He is embarrassed about this, and his relationship with his wife of 40 years is beginning to suffer.

Many people think that only women have issues with body image. But men have the same issues, too, and for many of the same reasons. One of the greatest challenges of living with an ostomy, an artificial passage into the body through which urine or feces is collected into a bag on the abdomen, is learning to live with an altered image of one's body. This may affect a person's self-esteem and sexual self-image in a significant way.

From Bob's experience, you will learn
- How body image may be affected by cancer surgery
- How this affects one's primary relationship
- How to deal with a stoma when sexual activity is planned.

Bob's Story

Bob is a retired factory worker. He is married to Jeanette, and they have three grown children. Bob worked in the same factory as his father did, and like his father, he was diagnosed with bladder cancer the year he planned to retire. Thirty years before, his dad didn't have much luck; he died within months of being diagnosed. There was always talk in the factory about safety and the chemicals they worked with, but there was work to do, and at the time, they really didn't think about what could happen many years in the future. When his dad was diagnosed with bladder cancer, Bob did stop and think a bit, but he had a young family to support and it was a good job, so he just kept on at the factory.

A year ago Bob went for his annual checkup, and the doctor decided to do a test on his urine. He had been getting up many times during the night to pass urine but thought this was just what happened when you got older. He was surprised when he received a call from the doctor's office asking him to come in again. The doctor explained that there was some blood in his urine and he needed to have more tests. Bob was a little confused by this because he didn't see anything in his urine, but he went to see the specialist.

The specialist wanted to do some tests. Bob wanted to get it over and done with, so he agreed to do the tests right then and there. Jeanette was waiting for him, and he asked the nurse to go out to tell her what was happening. She was shocked that he needed other tests but told him to go ahead and do it. The doctor passed a tube into his bladder and took a look and some scrapings. It was not a comfortable procedure, and Bob was glad he hadn't known ahead of time what would happen. The doctor told him that his bladder didn't look normal inside but that they would have to wait for the test results to know for sure. Bob left the office very subdued. Memories of his father and his swift decline filled his mind as he and Jeanette drove home.

A week later he heard the words he was dreading: He had bladder cancer and would need surgery. The specialist said that he had to remove the bladder completely and that Bob would pass his urine into a bag on the outside of his body. Bob didn't ask many questions. He agreed to have the surgery as soon as possible. Jeanette was very worried about him; he was quiet and seemed depressed. He didn't want to talk about anything related to the surgery and just wanted to get it over with. He made her promise that she would not tell their kids, who all lived in different cities. This was hard for her, but she agreed in order to make him happy.

Three weeks later he had the surgery. He was in the hospital for almost a week, and Jeanette spent most of the day at his bedside. He had a lot of pain in the first few days and slept most of the time. But she sat and waited for him to wake in case she could do anything for him. He was still noncommunicative when he was discharged, and the first week at home was a difficult one. He wouldn't let her help him with anything, but he sure seemed to need help. After a week when he did not shower and barely ate, she called their son Bobby who lived about three hours away. He drove down the following weekend.

Bob was both furious with Jeanette for calling their son but also very happy to see him. Bobby, had not followed his dad into the factory and instead was a high school basketball coach. As the oldest of the three kids, Bobby had a special relationship with his dad, and it was for this reason that Jeanette had called him. The two men sat outside on the deck for hours that first day. Jeanette peered through the window to make sure that Bob was okay. She could see them talking, although she couldn't hear their words. Bob seemed in a better mood later that day and into the next. He was quiet again when Bobby left for the drive back home, but he seemed to be making more of an effort to eat at dinner that evening.

Dr. Katz Explains

Take-Away Points

Everyone responds differently to health challenges. Bob has been diagnosed with the same cancer that killed his own father, and this may be something he had feared. They both worked in the same factory and were exposed to chemicals, a known risk factor for the development of bladder cancer. Like many men, Bob did not talk to his spouse about what was going on and just wanted to get the whole ordeal over with as quickly as possible. And he also asked his spouse to not tell their adult children about what was happening. He may not have wanted them to see him in what he perceived to be a weak condition. But in telling his spouse not to tell them, he deprived her of a vital form of support that she needed while he was having the surgery. Eventually she told one of their children, who immediately came to provide that support, more for his father than his mother.

- When there is a family history of a certain cancer, people often assume that what happened to parents or siblings will happen to them.
- Your family member's cancer and experience may be different from yours; treatments change and improve over time.
- Allow your family to support you. They feel helpless when they don't know what you are thinking or feeling.

Getting to the Root of the Problem

In the ensuing weeks, Bob got stronger every day and their son Bobby called almost daily. Jeanette could see his mood improve after he talked to Bobby, and once he even almost thanked her for calling him to come down on that weekend. Soon it was time for his follow-up appointment with the surgeon; it had been six weeks since his operation, and this was the time when they would learn about the success of the surgery from the pathology report. Bob was once again very quiet in the days leading up to the appointment. Jeanette knew it had something to do with his father but he would not talk about it. "Let's just get this over with," was all he would say when she dared to ask how he was feeling. She stopped asking after the third time he rebuffed her. This really was no different from how he usually behaved when it came down to talking about feelings; he didn't like to talk about the "mushy" stuff, as he called it. When he proposed marriage to her many years ago, it had hardly been romantic, so why would she expect anything else?

He hardly spoke at all on the way to the doctor's office. They waited only a few minutes before they were called. The specialist was waiting for them in his office, and Jeanette was glad that they were not in an examination room. The doctor got right down to business with very little time wasted: The surgery had been a success; removing the bladder had gotten rid of all the cancer, further treatment was not needed at this time, and because the erection nerves had been spared, Bob should not have any problems in that department. They were asked if they had any questions. Jeanette was so relieved that she had to try hard not to cry. She shook her head in answer to the doctor's question, and Bob got up from the chair. He seemed to be in a hurry to get out of there, and she followed him to the car.

Jeanette talked all the way home. She was so happy that everything was okay that it barely registered that Bob was not answering her. As they pulled into the driveway, she stopped and asked him what was the matter. To her surprise, Bob started crying. And not just a sniffle, either. He was sobbing like a child. The last time Jeanette had seen him cry was after his father's funeral. But now he was crying openly, his chest heaving. Jeanette sat there. She wasn't sure if she could put her arms around him, so she rested her hand on his knee. After five minutes, an eternity to her, he stopped. He wiped his face on his sleeve and stared out the windshield of the car. She instinctively knew not to say anything and instead they sat there, silent.

Jeanette waited until he seemed calmer, then she asked him what was going through his head. He answered her quietly and told her that he was sure he was going to go the way his father did. He had been praying for the last couple of weeks to hear good news from the doctor today, and he just couldn't believe that perhaps things would be better for him. He wanted to be sure that he had heard the same thing that she had; was it true that the cancer was all gone? Jeanette repeated what she had heard the doctor say. The cancer had been contained in the bladder, there was no spread, and everything looked good. She felt the tension evaporate from the stuffy air in the car, and they got out and walked toward the house. She went to call Bobby. He was waiting to hear the news from their appointment today and would be so relieved to hear that the news was good.

Dr. Katz Explains

Some people find it really hard to express their feelings, especially when they are afraid. Often, this feels like we are shutting out our partners from our lives and thoughts. We all have different ways of coping with challenges in our lives. In this case, Bob had held everything in. He was very afraid that what had happened to his father would happen to him, that the outcome of the cancer would be an early death. But as was mentioned earlier, your outcome will not necessarily be the same as a relative's cancer and its outcomes.

Take-Away Points

- Always take someone with you to medical appointments, and ask that they be present when you are given test results or instructions about procedures, medications, or treatments.
- You may want to ask that person to take notes, or even ask the healthcare provider if you can record the conversation so that you can listen to what was said over again to make sure that you understand what was said to you.

When Bob finally disclosed his feelings to his wife, it was as if a dam had burst. This is also not unusual; you can only keep fears and bad feelings contained for so long. Eventually they find a way of coming out. When Bob asked his wife to repeat what the doctor had told him, he was doing something very important. He was making sure that he had heard right. When we are hearing vital information, particularly when it relates to health or the outcomes of treatment, sometimes we don't hear everything exactly as it was said. That is why it is important to always take someone with you to medical appointments. You can't be sure how you will react to the information from the doctor, and that second set of ears will provide you with validation and clarification.

Men Can Be Mysterious Too

Things went back to normal in the next few months. Bob started doing his woodworking again, and Jeanette had a "honey do" list—a series of projects that she wanted her "honey" to do. He repaired the storm windows so that they would be ready to be put in place in the late fall, and he even went fishing with the neighbor once or twice. Jeanette had noticed that he wasn't as affectionate as he used to be, but she put that out of her mind. He seemed so much better. Perhaps she was just imagining things.

But when she did think about it, she realized that not only was he less affectionate, but also they had not made love since before the surgery. This was unusual. Bob had always had a strong sex drive, and at times she had found his demands to be too frequent. Over the past 10 years, things had really slowed down, but he still liked to try his luck once or twice a week. But now that she tried to recall, there had been nothing for many months. She remembered the surgeon saying something about nerves and erections, but she had forgotten the details in the time since that appointment. She decided to talk to him about it that evening.

Bob came in from his garage as the sun started to set. He washed up and was just about to pour himself a glass of beer when Jeanette came up behind him and slipped her arms around his waist. Never in a million years did she anticipate his response. He pulled away so fast and with such strength that she almost lost her balance. They stood about 10 feet apart, both of them out of breath from emotion. "What did I do wrong?" cried Jeanette. "What can I do right?" She started to cry, and Bob reached out for her. But he didn't enfold her in his arms as he usually would have. He held her almost at arms' length. Jeanette did not feel comforted. "What is wrong, Bob? Why can't you hold me?"

Bob let go of his wife and walked out the room. But Jeanette followed him, crying and pleading for an explanation of what had just happened and what was happening in their lives. "I am not letting you get away with this, Bob. You owe me an explanation. I cannot go on like this. Tell me what's happening!" She could see that he was struggling for the words. Talking had never been easy for him, but he could see she was not giving up. He sat down heavily in a chair. Looking at his hands, which were clasped together in his lap, he started to talk.

In a shaky voice, fighting back tears, he told Jeanette that he was afraid of what she would say when she saw his body. He had pulled away from her when she put her arms around him because he was afraid she would feel the bag attached to his abdomen. Jeanette listened in stunned silence. What was he talking about? After a few sentences, he stopped talking but did not raise his eyes from his lap. Jeanette was thinking as fast as she could. And then it became clear to her: They had not really touched since his surgery, and she had not seen him without his clothes on since then either! It all made sense to her now, and she knew she had to tell him that it didn't matter. But she was not sure that he would believer her.

Dr. Katz Explains

Take-Away Points

It is not unusual to feel shy about showing your altered body to your partner. You may not be sure what the reaction will be, and many people hide from their partners and avoid touch out of fear of a negative response. Some partners may, in fact, respond with some degree of shock; most of us have never seen a stoma, or opening on the skin of the abdomen through which urine passes. It would be helpful to see photographs of this before one goes through surgery to prepare for this, but this does not always happen. So seeing the stoma on your own body can be a shock, and some people feel sickened or even disgusted by what they see. Other people are more accepting and are able to be open about this. We are all different.

- If your surgical treatment involves the creation of a urostomy, ask the surgeon if he or she has photographs of what it will look like after the surgery.
- Preparation for living with a stoma is an important part of coping afterward.

Hiding

Jeanette tried her best to convince Bob that she was not going to reject him because of his urostomy. But her words sounded hollow even to herself. Could she really promise that she would be accepting of what she would see? Part of the problem was that she didn't know what to expect. The more she thought about it, the clearer it became how he had been hiding over the past months. He closed the bathroom door when he brushed his teeth at night before bed and emerged from the bathroom in his pajamas. And that was something else—he used to sleep naked in the summer and in a T-shirt in the winter, but he had taken to wearing flannel pajamas since his surgery. And he hardly ever wore a T-shirt around the house anymore. Even on warm days he wore those flannel shirts that he used to take on his camping trips. They were big and baggy, and he was obviously wearing them as camouflage. Her heart swelled in sympathy as she thought about the great lengths he had gone to in order to keep her or anyone else from seeing the bag.

Dr. Katz Explains

People often go to great lengths to disguise the bag with baggy clothing. And preventing oneself from being seen naked is another common strategy, with closed doors and dressing and undressing in private. Bob has obviously gone to great lengths to keep Jeanette away from the truth of what his body now looks like. This may not be necessary, but in his mind, he fears that she will reject him. This is not a rational response but a very human one.

Boys With Bags

Jeanette tried to tell him that she loved him no matter what changes his body had gone through. But she could tell by the way he held his shoulders that her words were not getting through. He looked defeated, which was something she had never seen before. Later that day, she was tidying in the TV room and found a bag of pamphlets and papers that Bob had received while he was in the hospital. He had obviously dumped it when he came home the first day, and it had lain there ever since. She started to look through the papers. Most of it was information about living with an urostomy and where to buy supplies, but there was also a pamphlet from a support group for people living with stomas. Maybe Bob could talk to someone like him who had also gone through this! Maybe that would help.

She tried to formulate a strategy to introduce this idea to Bob. She knew he was not going to jump at the chance; he was a very private man. But she felt in the pit of her stomach that this might help. Eventually she just blurted it out over dinner two nights later. "Bob," she started, "I want you to just listen to me and keep an open mind. I can see how you are struggling with this bag business, and I can't help you with that. But someone who is in the same situation can. There is a support group that meets at the hospital every month, and the people who go to this group have been through the same things you are going through. Can you go to just one meeting?" As she predicted, Bob's response was swift and final. "No way, no how, Jeanette!" But Jeanette had another suggestion: Would he speak to someone from the group in private, maybe on the phone? He seemed more amenable to this idea, and the next morning she called the contact person listed on the pamphlet.

A gruff male voice answered the phone, and Jeanette briefly explained why she was calling. The man, who introduced himself as Charles, listened to her story and then asked if her husband was available to talk right then. She was a little surprised by this and not sure how Bob would react, but she called out to Bob and asked him to come to the phone. She handed the receiver over to him and quickly left the room. She waited in the kitchen, fully expecting Bob to end the phone call within seconds. But the minutes went by, and she could hear his voice in the other room. Twenty minutes later he approached her, the phone in his hand. "Sounds like an okay guy," he muttered. "Going to meet up with him and some other people tomorrow for coffee." Jeanette just stared at him. She had certainly not anticipated this!

The next day, Bob went off to meet Charles and the others. They turned out to be three men of about his age, all of whom had some sort of bag like Bob's. Charles had also had bladder cancer, and the others all had colon cancer. Charles introduced Bob and told them that Bob's wife had been the one to call. This brought on a burst of laughter as they started to talk about their own spouses and their attempts to help. Bob listened in amazement; how could they joke about something so serious? One of the men, a tall fellow who looked like a stereotypical cowboy, seemed to sense Bob's confusion. "Listen, Bob. If you don't laugh, you cry. And life's too short to spend it sniffling and whining. So I crap out my stomach! It hasn't stopped me from doing the things I like to do, and the old lady still thinks I've got it!" Once again the others erupted in laughter.

One by one they told Bob how they came to accept what had happened to them and how they had learned to laugh at what happens, even when it was difficult. "We even have a name for ourselves," said Charles. "We're the Boys With Bags. A special group. You can join us if you want."

Take-Away Points

- Someone who has gone through a similar experience may be able to provide you with support, information, and encouragement.
- A local support group may be a good place to start.
- Go to one meeting and see if you are interested in attending any more—you may be surprised at what you learn!

Dr. Katz Explains

As much as family and friends can try to support and help you, it is really only someone else who has gone through something similar who can give you advice. There are support groups in most cities and even in some smaller communities for many different kinds of cancers. Some are open to both men and women with a particular disease, whereas others are gender specific or even age specific, with groups for younger adults and older adults. Some support groups have a professional facilitator, often a social worker or nurse from the local cancer center or the American Cancer Society. Other support groups are peer-led with one or more people from the group taking responsibility to organize and facilitate meetings.

But some people just don't like going to a support group. They may have a preconceived idea of what happens there, or just are not the kind of person who is interested in that format for support. There are other alternatives. You may be more interested in speaking to an individual who has had the same kind of surgery as you. It is often possible to be put into contact with an individual through either a support group or an association such as the United Ostomy Associations of America (www.uoaa.org). Or your physician or nurse may know of people who would be willing to talk privately to you.

Baring It All

Bob joined the Boys With Bags, as they referred to themselves. In just two weeks he found himself feeling very comfortable talking to them and was participating more actively in their noisy discussions over coffee each week. One of the men, Joe, had recently started dating a much younger woman. Bob asked him how he felt about her seeing him naked. Joe's answer was simple: If he didn't act like he was embarrassed or ashamed, then she would just accept it. The other men nodded in agreement. Charles described how he had gotten all worked up when he first took off his shirt in front of his wife, and her comment had been that nothing else of him looked like it did 40 years ago, so what was the big deal? Teddy, the last member of the group, agreed. His wife had been treated for breast cancer, and even though she had one breast now, she was still the same woman he had loved for more than 35 years. The men then told Bob how they managed with their bags during sexual activity. Charles wore a cummerbund to bed, and he had a whole collection in different patterns and colors to reflect his mood. The cummerbund anchored the bag and disguised the contents. Ted was able to remove his bag completely and seal the stoma itself with a plug when he made love to his wife. Bob was astounded at how much detail his new friends were giving him.

Dr. Katz Explains

There are many different ways to deal with the ostomy bag, and everyone has different issues that are important to them. Different kinds and sizes of bags are available, as well as caps that can be used to seal off the stoma for a short period of time. It may be as simple as emptying or changing your bag before sexual activity. A cummerbund can be helpful in anchoring the bag and preventing it from slipping or opening during sexual activity. Some men prefer to hide their bag, but you don't have to wear a baggy old T-shirt; a silk pajama shirt may make both you and your partner feel much more special.

Take-Away Points

- Ostomy therapists are specialized healthcare professionals, often nurses, who have a range of devices, tips, and strategies to help you deal with living with an ostomy bag.
- Your local ostomy association will be able to refer you, and many hospitals have ostomy therapists on staff as well.

Another Chance

Bob thought about this conversation long after it was over. Perhaps he had not given Jeanette a chance. He had told her that spending time with these men was helping him, but he had not really shared much about what they talked about. But he realized that he needed to talk to her more. So, that night after dinner he made some coffee and asked her to join him on the deck.

Hearing the other men talk so freely had given him some of the words he needed in order to talk to his wife. He started by telling her what they had disclosed to him. It just seemed easier to share their experiences than to talk about himself. But Jeanette quickly got the picture, and she gently asked him if he was having some of the same issues as they were. With a sigh of relief he admitted that he was ashamed of his body, was afraid of how she would react if she saw the bag, full of urine, just hanging there. And just like Teddy's wife, Jeanette told him that neither of them looked the same these many years later. But she hoped that he loved her the same way she loved him. A deeper love based on shared experience and children and growing old together. For the first time in many months, Bob took her in his arms and held her really close. He had another chance.

CHAPTER 7

Incontinence

I feel like a baby. Who needs this?

One of the most common side effects after radical prostatectomy is incontinence. This usually resolves over the months following surgery, and almost all men have control back by one year. Some men report that they are dry most of the time, but if they cough, laugh, sneeze, or move suddenly, they have a small amount of leakage. But this leakage can occur at any time, and it is not unusual for a man to leak urine during sexual activity. This can be devastating for the man and his partner, and one or both of them may feel disgust when it happens.

Marty has struggled with incontinence for the past year following his surgery. He has to wear pads every day to protect his clothing but has gotten used to this. What he cannot adapt to is the leakage that occurs when he is sexually aroused. Marty now avoids sex, and it is causing Lisa to feel rejected and unloved. She has tried to fix this but has failed and is very unhappy.

From Marty's story, you will learn
- How for some men, incontinence persists long after prostate cancer surgery
- How incontinence with sexual arousal can be bothersome
- What strategies can be tried to fix this.

Marty's Story

Marty's mother used to tell him that he was one of the lucky ones. He was always smart at school and popular, too. He was not drafted into the army during the Vietnam War because he had asthma, and he went to school and studied to be a dentist. He decided to specialize in children's dentistry before it became really popular, and he has made a very nice living in southern California. His wife, Lisa, is an accountant. They have three grown daughters, all married and living close to their parents.

Marty questioned his lucky life when he was diagnosed with prostate cancer at the age of 58. But his doctor, one of the best urologists in the area and a personal friend, told him he was still lucky; his cancer was small and the surgery would take care of everything. He was partly right. Marty recovered from the surgery quickly and was back at work within a month. The pathology report stated that the cancer was contained in the prostate, and Marty was pleased that he had chosen to have the surgery.

But as the weeks and then months went by, Marty grew more and more frustrated with the amount of time it was taking for his bladder to get under control. His friend the urologist told him not to worry, that for some men it just took longer. Marty was wearing pads day and night, and he tried to be patient. There were times when he thought things were getting better. He and Lisa went to Hawaii to celebrate their anniversary six months after his surgery, and he had only a little leakage every day. He thought perhaps he had finally turned the corner. But when they got back home and he went back to work, it was as bad as ever. He had learned to live with it, but he was not happy and thought ruefully that his luck had perhaps run out.

Dr. Katz Explains

Incontinence is a very common side effect after radical prostatectomy for the treatment of prostate cancer. After the surgery, one of the valves that stops and starts the stream of urine does not work properly. This is called the external sphincter, and it is located around the urethra at the level of the pelvic floor muscles. This sphincter doesn't work properly to prevent the flow of urine, so leakage occurs. This usually gets better over time, and less than 5% of men will still have significant problems with leakage one year after surgery. Anything that increases abdominal pressure, such as coughing, laughing, or sneezing, can cause leakage.

One of the factors that can increase leakage is fatigue. Marty noticed that when he was on vacation he had less leakage, but when he went back to work, it was bad again. As a dentist, Marty is on his feet a lot. This causes fatigue in all the muscles of his body, including the muscles of the pelvic floor, which help to keep the external sphincter closed. Alcohol also affects urinary control. Alcohol is a diuretic and therefore causes the body to produce more urine. It also irritates the bladder as well as relaxes the pelvic floor muscles, thus leading to leakage.

The Other Taboo

About four months after his surgery, Marty was a little surprised to see that his erections were coming back. He had spoken to a few acquaintances who had prostate cancer, and they all told him that after the surgery, his sex life would be over. At 58 years of age, this was not something that he wanted to hear. He talked to his surgeon about this and was assured that the erectile nerves would be spared and that the surgeon's rates for return of erections were among the best in the state of California. Marty didn't want to argue, and his mother had always said he was one of the lucky ones.

She was right, in part. As the months went by, his erections came back. They were not as firm as before, and if he was even the tiniest bit tired, he would not be able to get one. If he had even one beer or a glass of wine, they were not reliable, so he had learned to hold off on the alcohol if he and Lisa were thinking about having sex.

But while that was working well, there was something else that was not. When he became aroused, he leaked urine. At first he put up with it and found ways to disguise it. He kept his underwear on until just before penetration, and the fabric would soak up the leakage. Sometimes he would ask Lisa to join him in the shower or the hot tub because in the water the leakage would not be noticeable. They were not having sex all that often, so these strategies helped. He was not sure if Lisa noticed or not because she didn't say anything.

Dr. Katz Explains

Although Marty's progress with erections is good, his continued lack of continence is more challenging. Leakage of urine can happen when one is sexually aroused because this also causes the muscles of the pelvic floor to relax, which allows for some urine to leak. The amount of urine can be as little as a few drops and as much as a tablespoon or two. This can be very distressing for the man and also his partner.

Urine is sterile and does not do any harm if it touches either you or your partner. The issue with leakage at any time, but particularly during sexual activity, is a cosmetic one. Some people are bothered or even disgusted at the thought of this happening, and this can lead them to avoid any kind of sexual contact out of fear.

Marty has found a way to get around this. He invites his partner to join him in the shower or hot tub, where any leakage will not be noticed. A potentially less effective solution is his strategy of wearing underpants until penetration. Because they had never talked about it, he doesn't know if she has noticed or not. This could be seen as avoidance; he thinks she is okay with it and perhaps she is, or it may be that she does not want to say anything in case he hasn't noticed!

Take-Away Points

- If you have changed the way you have sex, especially after many years, your partner is going to notice.
- Not talking about what is happening never helps; it just creates barriers.

Cover-Ups

He had hoped that this leakage during sex would stop when he regained full control of his bladder, but it didn't. And he was still wearing pads every day. He managed this by focusing on how bad it would be to have accidents while at work. The thought of his patients or their parents seeing that was too horrible, so he rationalized the need to wear pads at work. He wore a cotton jacket over his shirt that covered his body to the top of his thighs, so he was sure that no one could see he was wearing a pad. Lisa told him he was being oversensitive and that you couldn't see anything even when he was wearing shorts and a T-shirt. He always wore his shirt untucked now and bought his clothes one size bigger so that his shirts and pants were baggy.

But as much as he covered up at work, at home there was less room to hide. As time passed with no improvement in his bladder control, he grew more and more despondent. Lisa noticed this change in him; he complained about being tired and often went to bed before her. When she got into bed he seemed to be sleeping, but there were times when she wasn't sure he was truly asleep and was instead pretending. She tried to talk about it with him, but he just rolled his eyes and told her she was making a fuss about nothing. He blamed his fatigue on being too busy at work, and yet he didn't seem to be doing anything about recruiting a new partner as he had planned to.

Lisa was increasingly unhappy about what was happening. One day as she was trimming the rose bushes in their garden, she found herself thinking about the last time they had made love. And she couldn't remember! She thought it might have been in the early spring, and here it was three months later and nothing had happened for all that time. She wasn't sure her memory was correct, so that night at supper she asked him. She thought she was sensitive in the way she asked, but Marty grew very agitated with her questions. "What difference does it make?" he shouted at her as he left the deck where they had eaten as the sun was setting. "That's gone now. It's over. Finished. I'm done!" Lisa was not sure why his response was so extreme. All she had wanted to know was if her memory was right and that it had been a long time since they made love. But he just blew up and walked off. The rest of the night was spent in silence. Marty watched television in the den, and she sat on the deck until it was time for bed. When she got there, he was lying on his side, facing the wall. She didn't try to talk to him or touch him, and as she went to sleep, she prayed that tomorrow it would be better.

Dr. Katz Explains

Not talking about the things that bother us in our relationships does not make them go away. Most of us know this through personal experience. Feelings, especially sensitive feelings, have a way of forcing themselves out of our mouths, usually in anger. That can lead to further bad feelings. Although Marty had been successful in covering up his need to wear pads in his underwear, he could not cover up what was happening in his intimate relationship. Every night he avoided his wife by either falling asleep before she came to bed or pretending to be asleep when she got there. He also blamed his lack of interest on fatigue from working too hard. When she asked him about the last time they made love, he blew up in anger. This kind of behavior does not resolve problems or allow couples to grow closer or understand each other better. It just leads to more hurt feelings and misunderstandings or even isolation if the partner also walks away.

A Desperate Woman

That night was the last straw for Lisa, and the next morning she decided to do something about what was happening. She had not slept much during the night, and she thought that Marty was awake a lot, too. But they had not talked or reached out for each other as they would have in the years before his surgery. They both lay there in the silence, alone.

Lisa made a plan: She belonged to the same book club as the wife of the surgeon who performed Marty's operation. They were not close friends at all, but Lisa was desperate and prepared to do anything to save her marriage. So she decided to call Lauren, the surgeon's wife, and ask to meet her. She thought that she might know how to deal with this situation given that her husband was a urologist. Surely they talked about things like this? Over the years Lisa had learned a lot about kids and teeth, so she was sure that Lauren had picked up some tips too.

Lauren seemed pleased to hear Lisa's voice on the phone and agreed to meet later that day at a coffee shop close to her home. Lisa was having some second thoughts about her plan as the day wore on, but she could hardly call and cancel at the last moment. Lauren arrived a few minutes after Lisa, and she had barely sat down before Lisa blurted out the whole story. Lauren was a little taken aback—this had never happened before with one of her husband's patients—but she tried to not let her facial expression give away her surprise. She really didn't know anything about what Lisa was telling her; her husband didn't talk much about work, and she liked it that way. So she waited until Lisa stopped talking and then in a sympathetic tone told Lisa that she needed to find help from a professional. She said she knew that her husband sometimes referred his patients to a sex therapist who worked in the same building, and she promised Lisa that she would pass on the therapist's phone number to her. And then they sat in silence, neither of them sure what to talk about after what had gone before.

Dr. Katz Explains

It is perhaps a measure of Lisa's desperation that she chose to seek help from the spouse of her husband's surgeon. There is no right or wrong in where you seek help. The important thing is to try and find help. People often assume that the spouses of physicians, nurses, psychologists, or other healthcare professionals know about the work that their spouse or partner does. Sometimes they do, but often they don't. Some people talk about their work at home, whereas others leave their work at the door when they get home. Spouses of healthcare professionals may know as little about the work that their spouse does as the next person. One thing that is important to remember is that a healthcare provider should *never* talk about specific patients at home or in any social situation.

Let's Begin

Later that day, Lisa checked her voicemail at home, and there was a message from Lauren with the name and contact information of the sex therapist as promised. Lisa was glad that she had not been home to answer the phone; she was feeling quite awkward about asking Lauren for help. But she knew they needed help, and she would do whatever she could to save her marriage. She really saw it that way. Something serious was happening to her marriage, and she wanted to fix it.

She called the number of the sex therapist right away, before she lost her courage. She had to leave a message, and within an hour, she received a call from a woman with a British accent. When the therapist, whose name was Dr. Bartlett, asked if Lisa would be coming alone or with her partner, Lisa hesitated and then replied that she would be on her own. They set up an appointment for one afternoon the following week.

Lisa did not tell Marty about her plans. She was still not sure that she needed to tell him. If she could fix things, then he didn't need to know. The following Wednesday she made her way to the building where both the urologist and the sex therapist had offices. Lisa was a little afraid that someone she knew would see her, but she passed no one on her way to the appointment. The therapist's office looked like any of the other offices in the building, with an ash-blond door and a discreet bronze nameplate. She entered a reception area that was decorated in gray and blue, and she waited as instructed by a small sign on the desk. Ten minutes later a tall woman with short black hair came through a door on the wall facing the couch where Lisa was waiting. She held out her hand in greeting and ushered Lisa into the room behind the door. This room looked very similar to the waiting area except that it held more furniture. "Let's begin," the therapist said in her crisp voice as soon as Lisa had sat down. "Tell me why you're here."

Lisa began to talk in a hesitant voice. She was not sure where to begin, and so she stopped and started in the telling of her story. Once or twice Dr. Bartlett had to ask a question to clarify something she had said, but she didn't interrupt more than that. When she felt she had told the whole story, Lisa stopped and was more than a little surprised when the therapist asked her how she was going to solve the problems she had identified. "Well, I thought that was why I was here," she stammered. "You're the therapist. Can't you help?" Dr. Bartlett smiled, and her face changed as she spoke. "I can only help the two of you to help yourselves. Your husband needs to be a part of this. When a couple has a problem, only the couple can solve it. You really do need to come in together." Lisa's face fell. How was she going to tell Marty?

But she knew she had to. Things were really tense between them. They had hardly even made eye contact since his blowup the week before, and she missed the way things used to be between them. Yes, they were husband and wife, but they had also been best friends, and that was what she missed the most. It was now a year since his surgery, and things were getting worse, not better. She had to do something.

That night after dinner, she asked him to go for a walk with her. The late summer air was filled with the smells of roses and barbecue as they strolled the streets of their neighborhood. Marty could sense that she had something to say, and he was afraid she was going to tell him that she was leaving him. He knew his outburst the other night was too extreme, but he was frustrated with what was happening in his life, so he lashed out at her. "I have something to tell you, Marty," Lisa said, "and you're probably going to get mad at me. Just let me talk, and then you can yell or not talk to me ever again. I went to see a therapist to talk about what I could do to fix what is happening between us. She said that we have to work this out together, that I can't fix it by myself. And there's another thing, and this is going to make you really mad. She's not like a talk therapist, she's a sex therapist. I'm sorry if that makes you mad, but I didn't know what else to do."

Marty didn't say anything for a few paces. He was not sure where to begin. He wasn't mad at her, but he felt shut out of his own life. He recognized that they needed to do something, in fact it was really he who needed to do something, but he was not sure that he needed to see a sex therapist! He could sense how tense Lisa was as she walked beside him, and he realized that he needed to say something. "I thought you were going to tell me that you were leaving me," he responded. To his surprise, Lisa started laughing. In fact, she was laughing so loud that a dog barked from behind a fence. "Leave you? Are you serious? Why would I leave you?" Lisa managed to say in between breaths. Her laughter rapidly turned into tears. "How could I leave you?" They stopped walking and stared at each other. "I guess we have a lot to sort out, a lot to talk about," said Marty, tears in his eyes matching those of his wife. "Let's see this therapist you've found. But I warn you, I am *not* having sex in front of her!"

Dr. Katz Explains

Many people have misconceptions about what sex therapists do. Lisa was embarrassed to be seen going into the therapist's office, and Marty thought he would have to have sex in front of her. Sex therapists are highly educated professionals who are experts in the study and treatment of sexual problems. They are also experts in helping couples find solutions to their sexual problems, which almost always involve problems with communication and other issues in the relationship.

Take-Away Point

- Sexual problems often are caused by communication and relationship problems.

Talk and Touch Therapy

One week later, Marty and Lisa went to see the sex therapist. He was a little surprised that her office was in the same building as his urologist, but he kept his thoughts to himself. They were greeted warmly soon after arriving and were shown into the office. Marty was not sure where to sit, but Lisa took his hand and sat down next to him on one of the couches. The therapist was the first to talk. "Lisa has told me what she thinks is happening in your relationship. To even the playing field a bit, let me tell you what I heard from her. Is that all right, Lisa?" Lisa nodded. She had not told Marty what she had told Dr. Bartlett, only that they had spent almost an hour together at that first appointment. "Lisa told me that she felt like she was being cut out of your life. That the two of you were drifting apart and that you hardly talked anymore. She also told me that there had been a fight when she asked you how long it had been since you last made love. She seemed to think that it had been a really long time, months, and she missed it and you."

Lisa was staring at her hands as they folded a tissue. Marty got the feeling that it was his turn to talk, and so he began, hesitantly at first but then the words just fell out of his mouth. Yes, it had been a long time, three months and two weeks in fact, but he was having this problem, and he didn't know what to do about it. Gently, the therapist asked him to describe the problem. "I leak," he said in a small voice. "Every time I get the least bit excited, sexually that is, I leak. It's disgusting, and I don't know how Lisa can even bear to think about making love with me." It was finally out in the open. Marty looked over at Lisa, not sure what he was going to see on her face. What he saw was pain and love and empathy. "I didn't know what was making you turn away," she said quietly. "I thought things were okay at first, after the operation. Your erections came back, and we made love a few times. But then it just stopped. And I didn't know why."

Dr. Katz Explains

It often is quite difficult to talk about sensitive topics, especially with the person whom you love most. But without talking, misconceptions can take over and build over time until your thoughts seem to be the whole truth. When a trained professional is in the room, many people find that it is easier to talk to each other than when they are alone. This may seem strange, but perhaps it's because there is security in knowing that an objective outsider will be able to control some of the emotions that may spill out.

A Helpful Suggestion

Dr. Bartlett allowed them to talk for a few minutes about how sorry they were for misunderstanding and making wrong assumptions. But she quickly brought the conversation into the present. "May I ask a few questions about this leakage, Marty? This is more common than you may realize, and I have a couple of things to suggest that may help." Marty nodded his head in agreement, and the therapist started to ask questions. He answered them as Lisa listened, her eyes growing wider as she heard how much this bothered him.

For the rest of the session, Dr. Bartlett and Marty talked about his incontinence. He didn't know that leakage with arousal and/or orgasm was fairly common, and he was surprised to learn that some of his attempts to hide this, like having sex in the shower or hot tub, were good strategies. She told him that something else that could work was for him to wear a condom during sex, but the look on his face told her that he didn't want to do that. She reminded him that emptying his bladder before beginning foreplay could also help, and they all laughed when he said that sex had better be quick if that was to work. "I have another suggestion that might work for you," she said as she reached into a drawer in her desk. She pulled out a small length of tubing that was folded back on itself. "This is a constriction band. Once your penis is erect, you place it at the base of your penis and tighten it. It is very effective for preventing leakage during sexual activity and has an added bonus of making your erection firmer and last longer." She spoke in a matter-of-fact voice and demonstrated how the constriction band worked over three fingers of her left hand. For the first time in a very long time, Marty felt like there was something he could do.

Dr. Katz Explains

For men who are able to have erections, using a condom to catch any leakage may be a good option. It will only help men who are able to have an erection because you cannot put a condom on a flaccid penis. But many men do not like using condoms or may never have used them and don't want to start at this stage of their life. The constriction band is an effective means of preventing leakage as well as helping to maintain the firmness of the erection. The band is made of latex and is placed at the base of the penis and tightened. It compresses the urethra inside

Take-Away Points

- Professional help can be of great benefit. Ask for a referral to a sexuality counselor or therapist who has experience working with men who have had cancer.
- If the therapist is helpful to you, tell your urologist and family physician so that they can help their other patients with such referrals.

the penis and prevents urine from leaking out. One type of constriction band is the Actis® (Vivus) band, which is available for purchase online.

Leakage with arousal tends to improve with time, and many men see improvement in the second and third year after surgery, so there is reason for hope. Currently, no medications are effective for this problem. Some men also find that pelvic floor exercises are helpful. Special physiotherapists can help with this. You can find a physiotherapist who specializes in this area by contacting the American Physical Therapy Association (www.apta.org).

Getting There

As soon as they got home from the appointment, Marty went to the computer to order the constriction band. He was pleased to see that it cost less than $20 because he was still a little skeptical that it was going to help. They had talked in the car on the way home about whether they would continue to see Dr. Bartlett. She had suggested that they continue to meet as Marty and Lisa work privately through their communication issues. Lisa really wanted to continue but Marty was less keen; he thought that now that he had a potential solution, they would be fine. It was just a matter of getting there. Only time would tell, but they had started on their way back to each other.

CHAPTER 8

Depression

A big part of me is gone.

Many couples and individuals mourn the changes in their sexual life and experience a range of emotions including anxiety, depression, and frustration because of the multiple losses experienced as a consequence of cancer and its treatments.

Roy knows that he should be happy to be alive; he had stage 4 melanoma, and his prognosis was not very good. But he has survived two years after surgery and chemotherapy, and everyone, including his wife, tells him that he should be happy to be alive. But he can't find a way to find the joy he once had in every day. Everything seems so black to him, and he can't find a way out.

From this story, you will learn

- How depression can happen long after treatment
- How treatment for depression can affect sexuality
- What alternative treatments for depression can be effective.

Roy's Story

Roy grew up one mile from the beach in southern California. He was one of those golden boys you see in commercials: tanned, windswept blond hair, big white smile. He surfed every day of his life even through college, and he found a way to stay outdoors when it came time to find a career. Roy worked for the parks department of his city, and most days he was outside, enjoying the sun as he went about his business, checking on the work crews.

He was always tanned, and over the years he grew quite vain about the color of his skin. Even though his wife, Susan, warned him about wearing sunscreen and a hat, he didn't listen. He had always been a sun lover. In his youth, had slathered himself with olive oil at the beginning of summer to ensure that he was the darkest one of the guys. He'd had a couple of bad burns back then, but he'd gotten over those.

Two years ago, Susan noticed that he had something on his skin, just under his armpit. Roy brushed her off; he hadn't noticed anything, but she persisted and pointed it out to him in the mirror. It was new and was about the size of a dime. What scared Susan was the color and shape; both were irregular, and as she looked at it, she got a sick feeling in the pit of her stomach. Susan had been a nurse for 25 years, and although she worked in the children's surgical unit, she knew enough that this mole concerned her. She insisted that he see their nurse practitioner about it and made an appointment for him immediately.

The next two weeks went by in a blur of unreality for Roy. The nurse practitioner took one look at it and sent him to see a surgeon in the next office, who did a biopsy. Three days later he heard the news: It was a stage 4 melanoma, and he needed more tests to see if it had spread. The next few days were a whirl of activity. He had a chest x-ray, a CT scan, and many blood tests. Finally, on the Friday of the second week, he and Susan met with the surgeon to review the test results. It was not good. The cancer had spread to his lymph nodes, and he had two spots on his right lung. He was going to need surgery, immunotherapy, and perhaps some radiation to the lung. Roy sat in the doctor's office staring out of the window. Every word the doctor said seemed to explode in his head, and he could feel Susan beside him, her body shaking as she tried to stop from crying.

When it was all over, he didn't remember much about the following weeks. He had the surgery to remove the cancer and was left with a large area under his arm that was just skin with no muscles underneath. It extended from just below his armpit to just above his waist and from under his shoulder blade to the front of his chest. It looked like a bad burn and was white and shiny. He could not look at himself in the mirror after his shower anymore. He had some radiation to his lung to kill the cancer that had spread there, and it seemed to work. He also had to have something called immunotherapy, which was supposed to help his body fight off the cancer. The injections themselves weren't bad, and Susan could give them to him at home, but they made him feel awful. He was really tired and felt like he had the flu most of the time.

Dr. Katz Explains

Melanoma is a serious type of skin cancer caused by exposure to the sun. Both long-term exposure and sunburns, particularly in childhood, are linked to the development of this skin cancer. Any change in an existing mole or development of a new unusual-looking growth on the skin is cause for concern. Treatment usually includes surgical removal of the growth and surrounding tissue but may also include other therapies intended to control the spread to other organs or provide relief of symptoms.

Out of Work and Out of Luck

He'd had to take off almost three months from work, and things were tight financially. He didn't want to burden Susan about this, but he was worried. Things were not good at work even before he had to take off time for his treatments. He was worried that he would not have a job to go back to. His boss had called a couple of times in the weeks after he found out about the cancer, but since then, he had not heard anything from anyone there. And one day there was a message from someone in the human resources department. They wanted to set up a meeting to talk about things.

Roy didn't say anything to Susan about the call. She'd been working extra shifts to earn more money, and he could see how tired and stressed she was. He felt bad about this; not only had she taken on the extra hours, but she'd also been his rock through all of this. She'd taken care of him after the surgery, given him the injections, and driven him to his radiation appointments, even when she was so tired from working the night shift that she slept in the car while he was having his treatment.

He went to see the HR director at the end of the week when Susan was working the day shift. He had a feeling it was not going to be good news, and he wanted to have time afterward to gather his thoughts before telling his wife. The HR director was professional, but ultimately the news was not good: They had to let Roy go. While he was away they had made some changes in the structure of the department, and they just didn't need him anymore. They had a check ready for him—six months' salary in a white envelope, and he was unemployed.

He drove to the beach after that and sat in his car, staring out over the water but not really seeing anything. His mind wandered to the years of his youth and the many hours he spent on this beach and many others like it. Things were simple then. What mattered most was the next wave, the next girl, the next adventure. He was so lucky then, and now his luck was gone. How was he going to tell Susan? He sat in his car for a while longer, trying to put off what he knew he had to do.

Susan took the news as he knew deep down she would. Her face paled for just an instant and then she literally shook her head, squared her shoulders, looked at him and said, "It will be okay. Trust me—we will make it okay." And for the most part, it was. Susan stayed on at the hospital but took a position where she worked the day shift from Monday to Friday. It was about the same money as her previous position but it was less tiring. She started selling a line of vitamins from home, and the work she did on that on the weekends helped a lot. Roy started doing some consulting work for a landscaping company, and for a while he enjoyed it. He applied for many other permanent jobs in his field but had little success with finding anything.

The Bottom of the Ocean

Over the following months, Roy grew more and more despondent. He felt like such a failure. Susan was holding things together, and he was contributing very little. Susan noticed that he was quieter and more withdrawn, but she was so busy at work and with her part-time sales work that she didn't say anything. He spent a lot of time sitting in his car, parked in a small parking lot overlooking the beach. It was winter now and every day there were surfers out there, waiting for the next big wave. From where he sat, they looked like small black birds, bobbing in the ocean. He could remember that feeling so well.

Without even realizing it, he got out of the car and started walking across the beach toward the edge of the sea. He still had his shoes on, and the wind whipped his jacket around his body. It was almost as if the waves were calling him, and he felt the water around his ankles, and then his knees. It was cold and it felt strange to be wearing clothes as he entered the water, but it felt right. A big wave knocked him off his feet. He stood up with some difficulty—his clothes were getting in the way—and he kept walking into the deeper water. He didn't hear the shouts of the surfers as they paddled toward him. It felt so good to be in the water again, like coming home. He felt the cold water fill his ears and then flow over his eyes, and then his feet lifted off the bottom and he was home.

The peace was disrupted by a pair of arms around his chest and a young voice close to his ears. "Dude, what're ya doing? You scared me, dude!" He tried to block out the words, and he struggled to get out of the circle of the strong arms and go back to the bottom of the ocean. But the young man was stronger than him and had more fight. Within seconds, a big wave pushed them toward the shore and they lay on the wet sand, both of them out of breath. The young man asked him his name, but Roy just lay on the sand, his eyes closed. The young man ran toward a pile of clothes behind a rock and rummaged in a bag until he found a cell phone. Within minutes the faint sounds of a siren could be heard.

Susan was waiting in the emergency department when the ambulance pulled in. Roy's cell phone was in his pocket but was ruined from the water. He had given the ambulance guys Susan's work number, and she had rushed downstairs to be there when they arrived. Her face was set in a grim expression but her eyes gave away the pain she was feeling. How could this happen to her golden Roy? To just walk into the ocean like that? To not even think of her and just want to end it all? She was sad and confused and hurt and afraid, and a little angry, too.

The nurses and doctors rapidly examined him and told Susan that physically he was fine. They had paged the on-call psychiatrist as was standard procedure for any suicide attempt, and they asked Susan to wait with her husband. She sat next to his bed where he lay with his eyes closed and his back toward the door. Her mind was full of questions, but she knew it was better to keep quiet and wait for the psychiatrist. The silence crept into her ears and entered her heart; it was the saddest sound she had ever heard.

Depression and Desperation

Within an hour the psychiatrist had spoken to them both privately and released Roy with the requirement that he be seen again two weeks later. He gave Susan the prescription for an antidepressant that he wanted Roy to take. "Fill that on your way home and expect some changes within two to three weeks," he said as he left the room. Susan drove Roy home. They stopped at the drugstore to pick up the medication, but they didn't talk in the car. Roy went straight to their room when they arrived. He didn't come out for dinner, and she left him alone. She knew she had to figure out her feelings before she could talk to him.

Susan spent a sleepless night lying next to Roy in their bed. He seemed to sleep—she heard him snoring off and on—but her eyes remained open in the dark. She had called the hospital when they got home and left a message that she was taking a few days off for a family emergency. By now most of the hospital probably knew their story—Susan's husband had tried to kill himself! He'd tried to drown himself and had been brought to the emergency department. She didn't really care who knew and what they thought. All she could think about was how it had come to this. He'd survived melanoma, for goodness' sake! Did he even know how lucky he was?

The next morning Roy came down to the kitchen just as Susan was pouring herself some tea. His hair was messy and for an instant he looked like he did when she first met him, young and a little shy. Even though she hadn't slept and was angry with him, she put down her mug and put her arms around him. She could feel his body relax as she touched his back and stroked his hair. He burrowed his face into the space where her neck met her shoulder, and she could feel his tears dampening her hair. "I'm sorry, Susie. I'm so sorry, Susie," he muttered. "I just feel so bad. You're doing everything and I'm doing nothing and I feel so bad." Her heart just opened to him. She could never stay angry with him for long, and he sounded so helpless.

And like they had done over the many years of their relationship, they forgave each other in bed. This was the way they had always resolved arguments, and it worked. Sex had been an important part of their relationship, and although it had changed over the years, they were still passionate about each other. It had been difficult after Roy's surgery and during his treatment, and then, of course, she had been working so hard. But they had always found a way to each other.

Dr. Katz Explains

Depression is quite common for people at all stages of the cancer journey. It may start at the time of diagnosis or during treatment. Many people are so involved in their fight against this disease that it is after treatment is over and when the fight is done that they become depressed. This can be very confusing: Shouldn't you be happy or relieved when you are done with treatment? Why would that be the time that you feel depressed? The reasons for this are many. When treatment is over, you actually have some time to stop and think about all that has happened. It may also be the time when you take stock of what physical changes have occurred. Once the busyness of having treatment is over, you have time to think, and this may be the time when the reality sets in.

Most people do not attempt to take their own life when they are depressed. But everyone is different. Roy didn't appear to plan what happened, and it almost seemed as if he didn't think about what he was doing and just walked into the ocean. He was lucky that someone was close by to rescue him and call for help. And if in fact this was a cry for help, it worked, and he was seen by a psychiatrist and prescribed medication.

One Step Forward, Two Steps Back

At the end of the second week, Roy was feeling better. He was actually quite amazed at how bad he had been feeling but at the time did not notice. He was sleeping better and had regained his appetite. He was also talking more, and he and Susan had talked about some of the things that had been bothering her about his behavior that she hadn't been able to talk about before. She told him that she felt rejected when he withdrew over the past months and also that she had been holding all the responsibility for their life without any emotional input from him. Roy immediately became defensive; he saw this as a criticism of his lack of employment. Before too long, they were arguing.

The fight did not last long. Within minutes Susan realized that her words had touched a sensitive spot for him, and she apologized. As was their pattern, they ended up making love on the couch in the den. It was like old times, but after a while Susan realized that something was different. Roy seemed to be having problems reaching orgasm. This had never happened before, and she was not sure what to do. Should she say something? What was he thinking? She was getting a little tired and sore, and yet he kept on. Eventually he stopped, and he lay down beside her. He was out of breath and his hair had turned brown with sweat. "Honey, what was that all about?" Susan asked. "I'm not sure," he replied. "This has never happened before. Sure feels weird though. What do you think?"

Susan took a few minutes before replying. She had read the patient education material that came from the pharmacist when he picked up his antidepressants. Roy had not read it, but as a nurse she always did. She had read that this medication could cause problems with orgasm. Just their luck! The medication had worked in so many ways. Roy was almost his old self, but he was also having one of the side effects. She knew she had to tell him, but part of her was afraid that he would stop the medication and get depressed again. Slowly she sat up and got dressed. "Let's make some tea and talk about this," she suggested.

Take-Away Points

- Don't just stop taking any medication without talking to your healthcare provider.
- Always ask if there are side effects from the drug you were prescribed.

Dr. Katz Explains

One of the side effects of the commonly used antidepressants in the selective serotonin reuptake inhibitor class (known as SSRIs) is delayed or absent orgasm. This is a side effect that is seen in both men and women. This side effect has led to these medications being used to treat rapid ejaculation in men; however, it is an off-label use (meaning it has not been approved by the U.S. Food and Drug Administration for this). Up to 80% of people on these antidepressants experience sexual problems as side effects, and many people stop taking the medication because they find the sexual side effects to be intolerable. There is variation in how badly people are affected, and some medications have fewer or more acceptable side effects. The risks of stopping the medication and not seeing a physician for another treatment are that the person continues to be depressed, and the depression may worsen.

A potential solution to this problem is to try another drug from this class, which may have fewer side effects or even improve things. Another antidepressant called bupropion (Wellbutrin®, GlaxoSmithKline) may cause few, if any, sexual side effects and can sometimes be added to another drug to treat depression. It has been reported that some people taking this particular drug actually experience improved sexual functioning including increased interest in sex, greater arousal, and more intense orgasms.

Self-Help

Susan made them some tea, and they sat out on the deck to talk about this latest challenge. She didn't want to have this conversation, but she knew she had to, and it had to happen now. "Honey," she began, "One of the side effects of the antidepressants you're taking is delayed orgasm. It's quite common, but I'm so sorry that it had to happen to you." Roy was characteristically blunt in his response. "Why are you sorry? You didn't do this. But I'm not taking any more of that crap. That's it. I'm done." Susan had anticipated this response from him. He would stop taking the medication and would get depressed again. She begged him to stay on the medication until they figured out something else. He agreed to stay on it for one more week.

She couldn't bear the thought of him being depressed again, so she did some research at the hospital. She talked to a few nursing colleagues and asked about alternatives to the medications for someone who was depressed. Two of these nurses suggested that she talk to one of the psychologists who worked in the employee assistance program. She called and asked for an urgent appointment; all employees of the hospital could access the services of this program for any kind of emotional support. She felt strange going to see the psychologist when she wasn't having a problem herself, but she didn't know what else to do.

She was lucky to get an appointment for the next day. The psychologist was a man about her own age who looked like a throwback to the '60s. He wore leather sandals and a colorful shirt with no tie, and his hair was tied back with what looked like a leather thong. Susan felt pressured to talk quickly, so she started by apologizing for taking up his time. Dr. Dave, as he asked to be called, told her in a calm voice that the next hour was hers, and she had no need to apologize. Susan took a deep breath and started again. She told him about Roy's problem. As she talked about it, she felt her face redden. She found herself apologizing for this too, and then laughed when she realized what she was doing. Dr. Dave was patient, and with a few skillful questions, he managed to lead her to telling him the whole story, starting with Roy's diagnosis. She told him everything—the surgery, the loss of his job, the suicide attempt, and finally the antidepressants and the sexual difficulty.

Dr. Dave asked her if Roy had followed up with the psychiatrist at the hospital. Susan's eyes grew wide with shock when she realized that they had not made an appointment to go back to see the psychiatrist who had prescribed the medication. How could they have forgotten that? The psychologist suggested that they do two things: First, Roy did need to see the psychiatrist again, and second, he offered Susan the opportunity to come back to see him regularly. Susan thanked him and said that her first concern was her husband but she would remember that she could come back to see Dr. Dave again. As she left, she picked up a booklet that was lying on the table in the psychologist's waiting room. The pamphlet was titled *Dealing With Depression,* and Susan slipped it into her purse.

Take-Away Points

- Always make and keep follow-up appointments with healthcare providers.
- Write down any side effects, however minor, that you have noted. Having a list will help to ensure that your concerns are dealt with.

Dr. Katz Explains

There are different options for treating depression. Susan has been proactive in seeking help for Roy and also herself. It is really important to follow up with any doctor who has prescribed medication for you. This is especially important when medication is taken for the treatment of depression. Because many people stop taking the medication as soon as they start feeling better, or, like Roy, when they have unwanted side effects, maintaining contact with the prescriber is very important. Just because you are feeling better doesn't mean that the depression is over for good. Many people find that the depression returns quickly once they stop taking the medications.

Taking a Stand

Susan talked to Roy about seeing the psychiatrist again. He was not that keen and was most concerned that he would be put on more pills, and he was done with pills! Susan had read the pamphlet on depression from the psychologist's office, and she encouraged Roy to read it. She had found it helpful and thought that Roy might, too. He was reluctant, but when she threatened to read it to him, he agreed to read it before his appointment with the psychiatrist.

Susan arranged to take the afternoon off the day of his appointment and met Roy at the psychiatrist's office. Roy thought this was completely unnecessary, but

Susan was insistent. She wanted to hear what both Roy and the doctor said, and she had some questions of her own. The couple met in the waiting room and sat in silence, waiting to be called. Within a few minutes they were ushered into the office of a tall man with red hair and a full beard. Susan didn't think this was the same psychiatrist who had seen Roy in the emergency department, and she was right. The man introduced himself as Dr. Mann and explained that the original psychiatrist would not be seeing Roy, and he would be taking over Roy's care. He then started asking questions. Susan felt Roy begin to tense up. She knew what he was thinking: Why did he have to answer those same questions when he had answered them before? Why did he even have to be there?

Susan quickly took over for her husband. She explained that Roy had experienced an unexpected side effect of a sexual nature and that he wanted to go off the medication. Roy looked up sharply when she mentioned the sex part; he had no intention of talking about that to anyone, and she had just gone and said it out loud! Dr. Mann nodded and turned to Roy: "What exactly are we talking about here?" Roy didn't know what to say. Instead, Susan answered for him. She told the psychiatrist that he had delayed ejaculation when taking the medication, and she—no, they—wanted to know if some other treatment was available. She told Dr. Mann that she had read that talk therapy could be as effective as medication and without the side effects. She had also read that exercise could help. She finally stopped to take a breath, and Roy looked at her in amazement. She was really assertive! He had known she had a mind of her own, but this was something else!

Dr. Katz Explains

It is always a good idea to take someone with you to medical appointments, especially ones where you will be given information about your diagnosis or treatments. The person accompanying you can be more objective than you and may also be able to remember more details afterward, which can be helpful to you. Some physicians, including oncologists, encourage patients to tape record the appointment so that

Take-Away Points

- Four ears are better than two! Take someone with you to all your medical appointments.
- Ask if you can record the session with your healthcare provider.
- Repeat what the healthcare provider has told you back to the provider to make sure you fully understood the information.

you can go over the details afterward as often as you need to until you have absorbed all the information. A second person with you can also take notes that are useful to you to reflect upon.

Making Choices

Dr. Mann listened to Susan, nodding his head occasionally and taking the odd note. When she stopped, he remarked that Roy had a great advocate, and Roy had to agree. He was not sure he would have used the word *advocate* but rather *she-wolf* for her strength and commitment, but advocate sounded pretty good. Dr. Mann then laid out some options for them. Roy could stay on the medication and hopefully things would improve in the orgasm department. Roy started to speak, but Susan put a hand on his arm, and he closed his mouth and let the doctor continue. Another alternative would be for Roy to not take the medication on the weekends, and hopefully his orgasms would not be affected over those two days. Roy shook his head at this one, and Dr. Mann smiled and continued. He agreed with Susan's reading about talk therapy being as effective as medications, but not for all patients with depression. And there was also evidence that exercise could improve mood. So, Roy had some choices.

Immediately Roy ruled out anything to do with the medication. Susan was not so sure about this, but she recognized that this was something affecting Roy's body, and he should make the final decision. Roy told the doctor that he had agreed to stay on the medication until this appointment, and he would now like to go off it and try the talk therapy thing. Susan immediately offered to exercise with him. Roy couldn't help but laugh at the thought of his wife, this busy woman, finding time to exercise . . . but who was he to claim to know everything? She had sure surprised him today!

Dr. Katz Explains

As the psychiatrist stated, evidence has shown that talk therapy (or cognitive therapy, as it is called) can help people to deal with depression. Exercise, too, has been shown to be of benefit. But each person needs to be treated as an individual, and although it may work for some, it may not work for everyone. The important thing is for Roy to stay in regular contact with the psychiatrist and have regular assessments of his emotional state. It is also important for a person to believe that any medication he is taking will help, and taking something against your will is not a good idea.

Three Months Later

Roy had started seeing a psychologist who worked with Dr. Mann. At first he didn't think that talking was going to help, but he was surprised to discover that it really did. They talked about his cancer and what that meant in his life, and about his job and how losing that had affected how he saw himself. He was shocked to discover that he hadn't really worked through the whole cancer experience and had instead buried his worries about his health. He realized that he had always had a sense of himself as the primary provider in his family, and taking time off work during his treatment and then losing his job had made him feel inferior.

Susan had been faithful in her dedication to getting him to exercise more, and they made an effort to walk for at least an hour three times a week. In that hour they talked a lot about the changes they had both gone through. Susan told him that she felt proud of her ability to contribute to their life in a meaningful way. Roy admitted that he had mixed feeling about that, but he could joke about being a kept man. He was able to laugh again, and his mood was definitely better. His waistline had shrunk, and Susan teased him often about being as sexy as he had been when he was a surfer boy. Their lovemaking was better than ever. Roy liked to think it was because of his better physique, but Susan thought she knew the answer: He'd been to a dark place, and now that he was back in the light, life was brighter than ever. Happy endings do happen.

CHAPTER 9

Communication

I have this little problem . . .

Communication about sexual feelings is often difficult, especially after cancer. The challenges for the single cancer survivor are perhaps even more significant. When do you tell a new partner that you have a part missing, or that you can't father children, or that you've been treated for cancer?

John was treated five years ago for lymphoma with a stem cell transplant. That time was really rough, and his marriage ended almost a year to the day after his diagnosis. It was a while before he could even bring himself to think about dating again, but the kids are older now and he has met someone who seems interested in him. But how is he going to be able to explain to her about the cancer?

In this chapter, you will learn about
- Strategies to help with disclosure to a new partner about a cancer history
- How to deal with fears about reactions from a new partner.

John's Story

When he looks back over the past five years, John can't quite believe how far he's come. Five years ago he was diagnosed with lymphoma, and what followed was, at times, a nightmare. Within months of his diagnosis he had a stem cell transplant. The procedure itself was fairly simple, but preparing for it was anything but. John spent weeks in the hospital in preparation for the transplantation. His whole body was radiated, and he was given a toxic regimen of chemotherapy to kill the cancer cells in his body. Then the stem cells from a donor were infused into his body, and the long wait began while those donor cells took over.

The entire time he was in the hospital, he was in an isolation unit. When the nurses entered his room, they wore masks and gloves and special gowns to prevent him from being exposed to infection. He could see their eyes but not much else. They didn't linger in his room, either, but rather dealt with his IV or took his temperature and then left the room. His wife, Miriam, came almost every day when he was first admitted, but as the days went by she seemed to make more excuses. First she had a cold and had to stay away. Then she said it was too hard to see him so sick. And then she had another excuse and another. He was too sick at the time to do anything about it. When he started to feel better, he spent hours lying in bed, trying to figure out what was happening to his marriage. Their children were 10 and 12 at the time, and though he hardly saw them, they called every day and sent him videos and cards. They didn't say much about their mother, and he knew it was not right to ask them what was happening.

Two days after he left the hospital, Miriam told him the truth: She was leaving him. She said she had been unhappy for a long time, and his time in the hospital confirmed for her that she wanted out of their marriage. She was leaving and was not taking the kids. And she was gone. He found out a few months later that she had met someone when he was in the hospital and was living with him. It was over, and he was alone with two kids and a long recovery ahead of him.

Take-Away Points

- Some relationships are strengthened by a health crisis such as this, whereas others founder.
- Get counseling support if your relationship is in trouble.
- Don't blame yourself if your relationship fails; you did not cause the cancer.

Dr. Katz Explains

Not everyone behaves honorably when a partner has a health crisis. We like to believe that we will be supportive and understanding, but some people just can't do the right thing, and they leave. Or perhaps what happens is that the partner is lonely and not coping and looks and finds something with someone else.

Moving On

It took a long time for John to feel better. The first year after his stem cell transplantation was difficult both physically and emotionally. He did not go back to work, and in some ways, that was a blessing. He had time to try to figure out how to run the house and take care of the kids. He couldn't believe how much was involved in the day-to-day activities of two children. The boys, then 11 and 13, were good kids, but they were messy and noisy, and most of the time the house looked like a tornado had gone through it. They were also used to their mom doing everything for them, and John couldn't and wouldn't do the same. He expected John Jr. and Tim to clean their rooms and take turns cleaning the bathroom; most of the time this meant yelling at them to do their chores, and he hated that. But they had to learn to contribute, and in the beginning, he really didn't have the energy to do much.

But as they grew older, things improved. John went back to work. He felt like a different person than the one he was when he was diagnosed. He was 25 pounds thinner and felt years older. His colleagues at the graphic design firm were a casual bunch, and though they welcomed him back, it was soon business as usual. The first week he felt like a spare wheel; he was not involved in any of the projects they had going and wasn't quite sure what to do. But at the end of the week, the senior partner, Len, called him in and assigned him to a new project. He was back and was grateful he still had a job.

Dr. Katz Explains

The first year after a stem cell transplantation is often a very difficult one. Fatigue is a common side effect of the treatment, and the person who has received the transplant has to be very careful to avoid any kind of infection. This makes going to work challenging, and many transplant recipients don't go back to work until after the first anniversary of the transplantation. At this point, transplant recipients also receive all their immunizations again because the immunity that they had from childhood immunizations is destroyed by the radiation and chemotherapy.

Take-Away Points

- Ask for help when you need it. Asking friends and family to do specific tasks (like laundry or washing dishes) gives them something tangible that they can do.
- Grant yourself grace when you can't do something because you are too tired.

Life Goes On and On

Five years go by fast when you are the single parent to two teenagers. John Jr. was now 17 years old and preparing to leave home for college. He'd been accepted to a good school on a tennis scholarship, and John was so proud of him. He'd been difficult that first year after Miriam left and John was recovering from the transplantation. But he had matured a lot since then and was eager to leave for school and the adventures that would follow. Tim was now 15 and, like most kids his age, spent most of his time with his friends and not much time with his father. John knew this was normal; after all, he'd gone through this with John Jr., but part of him wondered what it would be like with just the two of them in the house.

John Jr. left at the beginning of August, and the house was really quiet. John took Tim on a camping trip. Although they had a good time, it was strange to be just the two of them. Tim was much quieter than his older brother, and John found himself asking his son a lot of questions to fill the silences. But they fished and hiked, and at night they sat by the campfire, watching the sparks explode into the dark. John didn't shave the entire week and was surprised at the end of the week when Tim's cheeks were covered in stubble, too—his little boy was not so little anymore! When they got home from vacation, Tim went back to his usual ways, asleep most of the day and out with his friends till the early hours of the morning. John felt like he was living alone, and for the first time in years, he was lonely.

Strangers in the Night

John liked the people he worked with at the graphic design studio. Most of them went out for drinks on Friday evenings, but he hardly ever went with them. It seemed more important to go home and make dinner for the boys. But now John Jr. was out of the house, and Tim was out most nights. So one Friday night, soon after the camping trip, John went out with his coworkers. Eight of them headed out for a bar close to their studio, six men and two women. They had finished a big project that week and were in a mood to let off some steam and have a good time. John couldn't remember having so much fun—well, at least not for a long time.

The bar was busy, and it took a while for them to find a table where they could all sit together. They ordered a pitcher of beer as soon as they sat down, and then another. Soon they were laughing and shouting over the other voices. Before long some of the people at the next table had joined in their loud conversation, and John found himself sitting very close to an attractive woman from the next table. He soon found himself talking to her despite the loud music. They managed to hear each other, although at times they had to use improvised signals to make themselves understood. After a while they both glanced at their watches at the same time, and laughed when they realized they had done this in unison. They stood up together, waved good-bye to their respective tables, and made their way through the crowds to the exit.

They stood outside in the quiet and dark. John was a bit embarrassed—what was he supposed to do now? The woman put out her hand and introduced herself as Michelle. "I'm John," he replied, feeling awkward. "It was nice to meet you, John," she replied. They stood there for a while, not talking but not making any move to leave. "Would you like to get a cup of coffee?" she asked. John laughed in relief; he couldn't believe how bad he was at this. He was 45 years old after all, but then again, he hadn't really talked to a strange woman, other than the nurses, in quite a while.

They walked down the block and found a coffee shop where they sat down after ordering tea. They both laughed about this; why weren't there tea shops for tea drinkers? Michelle was easy to talk to. She appeared to be in her early 30s, and she worked for a group of architects as a draftsperson. They had quite a lot in common, and their conversation flowed from one topic to another. Before they knew it, the staff started cleaning up around them. It was 10:30 pm already! John was surprised at how quickly the time had gone by, and he stood with her while she waited for a cab. He walked the two blocks to where his car was parked, his fingers touching the piece of paper where she had written her phone number and e-mail address.

The Dating Game

John called Michelle the next day. He thought it might be too soon, but he really didn't know the rules of the dating game at this point in his life. She seemed pleased to hear his voice, and they made plans to go to a movie Sunday night. They were both interested in seeing a movie at a small theater downtown that showed mostly arty movies—one more thing they had in common! The date went well. They ended up going out for dinner at a small bistro close to the movie theater. They lingered at their table long after the meal was finished, and once again the staff started cleaning up around them.

They shared some of their personal histories this time. Michelle had moved there to find work after college. She had never been married and lived alone with a 15-year-old cat that she had brought from her family home. John was not sure what to tell her about his history. He told her that he was divorced and that he had two boys. She seemed a little taken aback by that. He tried to make a joke about fathering the kids when he was really young, but that fell flat, so he just told her his age. She was 35 years old, and the 12-year difference didn't seem to bother her. But after that disclosure, John was not sure what else to tell her. He had not been in this situation before. How much of his medical history did he have to tell?

Take-Away Points

- Trust your instincts; you'll know when the time to tell is right.
- There's no right or wrong way to tell someone that you've had cancer. Take a deep breath, get the words out, and then wait for the other person to say something or ask a question.
- Don't give all the details at once. Start simply and see where things go.

Dr. Katz Explains

It's often difficult to decide when and how much to tell about your history. The timing is perhaps the most challenging part: too soon and you may think you will scare the person off, but if you leave it too long, will they think that you have hidden something? There's no perfect time to tell someone about your cancer history. But at some point, you should share this information. The time to do this is probably when it feels like the relationship is going somewhere. It takes courage. You may be really afraid of rejection, especially if this is the first person you have dated after your diagnosis and treatment. John and Michelle have progressed past the first date, so he should say something sooner rather than later.

Laying It on the Line

The next time they went out, this time for a walk around the lake near Michelle's house, John knew he had to say something. They were talking about their childhoods, and Michelle was describing the farm where she lived as a child. Her voice had a faraway quality to it as she talked about her parents, who came from a long line of dairy farmers, and her siblings. She hesitated when she gave their birth order, and then told him that her younger sister had died of childhood leukemia. John reached out and took her hand and the words came out: "I had cancer five years ago. I know this may be too much information, but I need to lay this on the line. If it's too much for you, with your sister and all, then we can just call it quits right now." Michelle stopped walking and stared off into the distance. John felt his heart beating in his chest like a bongo. The heartbeats seemed to count the seconds that she didn't say anything. And then she turned to him with a serious look on her face. "Thanks for being honest, John. I'm not sure what I feel right now. To look at you, no one would ever know that you'd been sick. But we do need to talk about this more. Not because I will judge you, but because I need to know what this means and what I'm getting myself into." She blushed as these last words came out; perhaps she had overstepped some boundary. Who knew if they were getting into anything? John led her over to a bench overlooking the still water of the lake. They sat down, and he started to talk.

> **Take-Away Points**
>
> - The perfect situation may just present itself, and that is the time to tell.
> - Don't overthink it. Talk from your heart.
> - Getting your history out in the open will allow for an honest relationship and takes away the fear of her finding out some other way.

The Whole Truth

John wanted to tell her everything, but after five years he was not sure that he even knew what "everything" was. His memory of the time he spent in the hospital was colored vividly by what happened with Miriam, and he couldn't think of that time without feeling betrayed by her. His memories of the year after the transplantation were clouded in the fog of exhaustion of caring for two young boys alone, overlayed by his fatigue from the recovery process. Everything was so complicated!

As he answered her questions and tried to remember what the experience had been like, he felt strange that she was the first woman he had talked to about this. In fact, this was the first woman that he had spent any time with since his marriage broke up. As he thought about it, he realized that this was the first time in five years that he had been interested in a woman! Five years was a really long time by anyone's standards. What was that all about? Michelle could see that he was distracted by something, and she assumed that he was having difficulty talking about his illness. She didn't want to pressure him, and so she let the conversation end. They continued walking around the lake. When they got to the parking lot, they wordlessly got into his car and sat in silence.

John's thoughts were focused on the long time in which he had been almost without any sexual thoughts or feelings. He saw it clearly now in retrospect. He had been living an almost totally asexual life! What did this mean? Michelle was not sure what to think. They had been talking, and then suddenly it was as if John just went away. They drove in silence, and soon they were outside Michelle's small house. She was not sure what to do—should she invite him in for a cup of tea, or was it better to just let him leave? John made that decision for her. He apologized to her and said he needed to get back home to spend some time with Tim. He seemed distracted, and she realized it was better to let him go and deal with whatever was bothering him than to prolong their date. She was sad, but this was only their second date, after all. She didn't know him that well, and perhaps she never would.

John drove home, barely seeing where he was going. He circled the block where his house was three times before he parked in the driveway. His mind was full of memories and confusion and concern. When was the last time he even thought about sex? Was he even aware of when last he had an erection? He knew that since he'd met Michelle he'd imagined what it might be like to kiss her, but was that all? What was going on? He didn't know where to turn, and he felt panicked about how he was going to sort this out. Suddenly he remembered that long ago, when he was preparing for his stem cell transplantation, one of the nurses had given him a package with all sorts of pamphlets. He hadn't bothered reading them at the time, but he didn't recall throwing them into the garbage. So maybe he still had them somewhere. He rushed into the house, past Tim who was sprawled on the floor playing a video game. He reached the office and started rummaging through drawers and bookshelves. And suddenly there it was! The package that the nurse had given him five years earlier was sitting where he had left it so long ago. He tipped out the contents, found a book, and started to read.

Dr. Katz Explains

John has been through a lot in the past five years. Not only did he have a stem cell transplant, but his marriage ended and he had to learn to take sole responsibility of his two sons. The first year after stem cell transplantation is usually quite difficult, and John not only had to cope with his health but also with parenting and household issues. John is not unlike many men in relation to how he dealt with the patient education material he received from the nurse: He ignored it! Everyone is different, and some men (and women) read voraciously and widely when they are diagnosed with any kind of illness. And others either leave the reading to their partner or don't bother with it at all. There are many houses and apartments where you could find packages of patient education material propping up bookshelves or lying in a deep drawer.

Take-Away Points

- Everyone's needs for information are different.
- Old material may contain old information. If you want to review something years after your treatment, you may be better off searching the Internet or contacting the hospital for newer information. But be careful about what you find on the Internet because not all sources are reliable.

It Says in the Book . . .

John read all the material in the package. One of the books was particularly helpful. As he read, he discovered that everything he had gone through, except for the part where his wife left, was explained clearly. Many of the symptoms described, he had experienced. One of the chapters was on sexuality, and he read that it was extremely common for men to have little to no interest in sex for a while after stem cell transplantation. It was like a light had been switched on for him! There were examples in the chapter from men and women who were having problems years after their transplantation, and though it made him worry about himself, he was also glad to read that he was not alone. The book recommended that transplant recipients who were having problems should contact their healthcare providers to find out if their hormone levels were normal. Without hesitating for a moment, John called the transplant coordinator at the cancer center where he had been treated five years ago. Nancy was the person who had helped him when he needed his transplant, and she was still working there. He had forgotten it was Sunday, so he was a bit surprised when no one answered and the voicemail message played.

He was so happy to hear her voice on the voicemail message and to not have to explain everything from the beginning to a total stranger. The next morning she called him at work, and he went to the cancer center at lunchtime to have some blood drawn for tests. He was not due for his follow-up appointment for a couple of months, and he really didn't want to wait until then.

This Explains It . . .

Three days later, he went back to see the transplant specialist to find out what the blood tests had shown. He had seen Dr. Shaw so many times over the years, but each time he was shocked at the sight of her; this highly qualified specialist looked like a 12-year-old. She was petite with long blond hair that she wore in a braid that reached almost to her waist. She had a broad smile with a gap between her two front teeth that reminded him of a naughty school kid. But she really knew her stuff and was very professional in her dealings with patients. He remembered her from his days in isolation when he had the transplantation. Her long braid barely fit into the cap that she wore over her head, and the gown looked like it was 10 sizes too big for her, which it probably was!

Dr. Shaw seemed pleased to see him and waved away his concerns about wasting her time. "Let's see what we have here," she said as she scanned the piece of paper with his blood test results. "Hmm, everything looks fine except that your testosterone is on the low side and your prolactin is high. This happens in men after transplant, and I'm not sure why we didn't pick this up sooner. This explains your symptoms. It's pretty easy to fix." John felt the air leave his lungs in a big whoosh. He wasn't aware that he'd been holding his breath, but now that he was breathing normally, he realized how anxious he'd been.

Dr. Shaw started to write a prescription for him and then stopped. "The first thing I'm going to do is give you some pills to drop the prolactin in your blood. Then we'll measure your testosterone again in a month or so. If your testosterone comes up, you'll be fine and won't need other treatment. If it doesn't then we'll need to talk about giving you some testosterone replacement. How does that sound?"

Dr. Katz Explains

Increased levels of prolactin cause a decrease in production of testosterone in many men following stem cell transplantation. The effect of lowered testosterone levels is often felt as fatigue and lack of interest in sex. Some men also experience erectile dysfunction as a result of this. However, these side effects may also be caused by the significant changes to normal life both during and after the stem cell transplantation. John's life was complicated by his wife leaving him for another man while he was recovering from his transplantation. Libido, or interest in sex, is not merely a hormonal issue but also involves our thoughts and feelings. John has shouldered many burdens alone since his treatment, and this may be playing a part in his lack of interest as well.

High levels of prolactin can be treated with a drug called bromocriptine. This drug reduces the amount of the hormone produced by the pituitary gland. Testosterone levels should rebound once the level of prolactin in the blood decreases, but if the level of this hormone remains low, testosterone replacement therapy may be started.

Take-Away Points

- Sexual difficulties are not less important than any other symptom.
- There may be a fairly simple explanation for what you are going through, but unless you ask about it, nothing can be done.

It's Getting Better All the Time

John noticed a difference within a couple of days. He was really tired and had been warned that drowsiness was one of the side effects, so he took some time off work. He napped when he needed to, but the rest of the time he did some house cleaning. And did he clean! He started in the office where he had found the package of information for his transplant five years ago. He filled six big garbage bags with stuff, a lot of it still from Miriam. There were old magazines and romance novels that went into the recycling box, but there was plenty that just went into the garbage. He needed a nap after that, but when he woke up, he started on the bathroom and then the bedroom. John Jr.'s room was pretty neat; the boy had cleaned up himself when he packed for college. Tim's room was another matter, but John wanted him to do it himself. At the end of three days he felt like a new man. But it was not just the cleaning that had done it. He really did feel like new, and in all sorts of ways that he hadn't thought about in years. He was thinking about Michelle a lot, and some of his thoughts were x-rated! He could hardly wait for that evening when he was going to call her to suggest a date the next night. Things were certainly getting better all the time.

CHAPTER 10

Fertility Problems

We were talking about starting a family when this happened.

Fertility issues are important to younger adults when they have to undergo treatment for cancer. They're often forced to make difficult decisions at a time when the threat to life is foremost in their minds. Simon had just gotten married when he discovered a lump in his testicle. He was soon diagnosed with testicular cancer, and now at the age of 27, they are unsure if they will ever be able to have children.

In the shock and terror of a cancer diagnosis, this young couple has to face some important decisions. Making a sperm donation will delay the start of his treatment, and is it worth it? His wife, Tara, tells him that it doesn't matter, but this was their life plan, and now it may be over.

In this chapter, you will learn about
• The importance of sperm banking
• The reality of the options for fertility preservation.

Simon's Story

Simon and Tara are in their late twenties and started dating when they met in college five years ago. Simon and Tara were both on the swim team, and their attraction was instant. They are both tall and athletic with the lean and long bodies of swimmers. Their friends would always tease them that they would have the best-looking kids, and they secretly agreed. When they realized that they wanted to spend the rest of their lives together, the thought of a bunch of blond children was part of their dream for the future.

Simon had started as an associate in his father's law practice, and Tara was continuing her education with a graduate degree in botany. They married on a beautiful summer's day in the Napa Valley. Tara wore flowers in her hair, and Simon was striking in a linen suit with a pale pink shirt that matched those flowers. The guests were slightly in awe of this beautiful couple and the promise of their life.

When they returned from their honeymoon, they moved into a condo downtown and started their new life together.

A Small Lump

One morning when Simon was showering after his run, he noticed a small lump in his testicle. He was a little distracted by thoughts of a meeting later that morning with a new client, and so he didn't think about it beyond a momentary prick of concern. The next morning it was still there, and this time when he went looking for it, he knew in his gut that he was in trouble. He called to make an appointment with his family doctor, and the first available appointment was not until the next week. He thought about saying it was an emergency but decided he could wait. He first needed to talk to Tara about this, and he needed to think about how he was going to do that. She was busy preparing for her dissertation defense, and he didn't want to stress her out any more than she already was.

That night in bed he told her what he had found. Her eyes widened in fear and she started to cry. He assured her it would be okay, but he knew he was lying. He was not sure that anything would be okay after this. The following Monday he saw Dr. Jones, who examined him and thought the lump was suspicious. He sent Simon to see a urologist the next day, and the urologist ordered an ultrasound of the testicle as well as blood tests. A sense of unreality settled over Simon. He hadn't told his father or mother about what was going on. He was worried that his father, the founding partner of the law firm, would notice his absences from the office. He just couldn't find the energy to exercise, and he mostly sat on the sofa at night, deep in thought. Tara was extremely anxious while this was happening. She wanted to accompany Simon to his appointments, but he wanted to go by himself. She tried to focus on her dissertation but spent most of her time staring into space.

The call from the urologist came late on Wednesday afternoon. He wanted Simon to come in the next day early to go over the test results. Simon had a sick feeling in the pit of his stomach. He told Tara that he wanted her to go with him to hear the news. Neither of them slept much that night.

Now What?

The next morning they arrived at the urologist's office and were seen within minutes of sitting down in the waiting room. Dr. Able ushered them into his office and got right down to the point: Simon had testicular cancer and needed to have the testicle removed. The young couple sat in stunned silence. Although he had prepared himself for this, Simon was not prepared for the icy cold waves that washed over his body. Tara was trying not to cry, and he could sense her reaction but could not bring himself to look at her. He needed to gain control over his feelings. He knew that he needed to listen to what was being said and to find a way to get through this. "When can we do this, Dr. Able?" were the first words out of his mouth. The doctor replied that that the surgery should happen within about a week but cautioned the young couple that they needed some time to talk about things. Tara was not sure what they needed to talk about. As Dr. Able gently explained about fertility preservation, Tara's heart sank. This might mean that they couldn't have babies. In that instant she realized that the dream they had had for so long—those blond babies—might have slipped out of their reach. In that same instance she realized that it didn't matter. Now what?

Dr. Katz Explains

Testicular cancer usually occurs in young men but can happen at any age. Treatment always involves surgical removal of the affected testicle, and radiation or chemotherapy may follow based on the kind of cancer. Although removal of one testicle does not mean that the man will not be able to father children, many men who have testicular cancer have problems with their sperm production even before the cancer is diagnosed. They may produce too few sperm, sperm that are misshapen, or sperm that don't move fast enough or move in the wrong direction.

We've Got to Hurry

Simon wanted to think about what Dr. Able had explained about fertility preservation. He prided himself on being a logical and rational person; he was a lawyer, after all, and a good one with a reputation among his peers for being analytical about everything. But now, when he most needed to think clearly, his mind was whirling in circles! Tara was crying, the tears running down her cheeks and onto the front of her shirt. He had never seen her cry this much, and it frightened him. Had he missed something the doctor said? He thought he heard that he would need surgery soon, but she was reacting as if he were going to die immediately.

He took a deep breath and asked the doctor outright was his prognosis was. "Pretty good if all goes well," replied Dr. Able in a calm voice. "We'll know more after the surgery, of course, when the pathology results will be in and we can tell what kind of cancer it is and if you will need any other treatment. I understand how difficult this is for you both. It's never easy, of course, but you are just starting out in life, and you have to make some important choices that will influence many other things in your life."

Simon felt his heart rate slow down a little. "When is the deadline to set a date for the surgery? How do I get more information about this fertility stuff? When do I have to tell you what I am going to do about the sperm banking, Dr. Able?" Simon seemed to have found the analytical part of his brain and was creating a list of what he needed to think about and when. Tara stared at him. "What are you talking about, Simon? What are all these questions? Just tell the doctor that you'll have the surgery immediately, and we'll worry about everything else later. We've got to hurry!" Dr. Able looked from one to the other and gently told Tara that Simon was doing the right thing. A day or two or even five was not going to matter, and the future of their family, by that he meant children, rested on the decision that Simon would have to make in the next few days.

Tara tried to tell the doctor that she didn't care about children, that what she cared about was her new husband surviving this cancer. But she was once again crying and couldn't get the words out. Dr. Able suggested that they go and talk to the fertility specialist as soon as possible. His receptionist would call the fertility clinic and make an appointment, perhaps as soon as that afternoon. With additional information about sperm banking and costs, they could perhaps speed up the process, and Simon could have surgery at the end of the week. Simon could see how Dr. Able was trying to find a compromise for Tara's sense of urgency and his own need to think this through as logically as he could. He thanked the doctor and led Tara to the waiting room. The receptionist had already made the appointment with the fertility specialist for 4 pm that afternoon. Coincidentally, the fertility clinic was in the same building as Tara's OB/GYN, and Simon knew that would be a challenge for his wife.

Dr. Katz Explains

It is always difficult making decisions that could affect your health for the rest of your life. It is even more difficult when the condition you have is potentially life threatening. It is also not uncommon for two people in a couple to have opposing views on what should be done, as was the case with Simon and Tara. She wants him to have surgery immediately and deal with any consequences later; she wants him to get rid of the cancer first and survive. Simon wants some time to consider what this would mean for their future; he is not focusing so much on the threat to his life but rather on the threat to their dreams.

It is always a good thing to take some time to make important decisions about treatment, as you have seen over and over again in the stories of the couples in this book. Although your natural impulse to do something *now* is very strong, taking some time, even a few days, to think about it is always better in the long run. Some people who do not have that time can have many regrets after treatment or feel angry that they didn't have choices or were told what to do, which can affect long-term quality of life.

Take-Away Points

- Even if your partner pressures you to act quickly, you should take as much time as you need to think things through and make decisions.
- Getting more information can be helpful in pointing the way to where you need to go, so ask if there are other specialists that can give you more information or support in this difficult time.

Just Tell Us What to Do

Simon and Tara didn't talk much the rest of the day. He called his office and said he had come down with the flu and that he wouldn't be in for a couple of days. He asked Sue, his secretary, to not say anything to his dad to keep him from mentioning it to his wife, who would then come over with soup or cookies. He tried to make a joke of it, telling Sue that Tara would be baking the cookies.

He hoped that it actually sounded like a joke because to his ears, it sounded desperate and terrified. He spent most of the day on the Internet searching for information about testicular cancer. He went to Lance Armstrong's LiveStrong Web site and was reminded of Lance's remarkable survival story as well as the stories of other cancer survivors. He felt his heart grow just that little bit more hopeful and tried to show Tara what he had found. But she was in part angry with him and in part almost hysterical, and he found for the first time in all their years together that he couldn't talk to her.

At 3:30 pm they set out to see the fertility specialist. They were early for the appointment, as the clinic was very close to their home, but Simon wanted to get out of the condo, and he needed to feel like he was doing something instead of just sitting around. As they entered the building, they saw one of their friends coming toward them over the marble hallway. Tara drew in a sharp breath—what was she going to say to her?—but the woman must have assumed that they were going to the OB/GYN and just waved and smiled at them.

The fertility clinic was even more luxuriously decorated than the OB/GYN offices, and Simon chuckled to himself that business must be good. They had to fill in many forms, which took about 15 minutes. When the receptionist saw that they were finished, she escorted them into an office toward the rear of the clinic. Dr. Forester was a young man, just a few years older than Simon, and he had a confident manner. Simon could tell he was used to dealing with stressed-out couples. He was calm and friendly and started off by acknowledging how difficult this must be for the couple in front of him. Tara was fighting back tears, and Dr. Forester moved a large box of tissues closer to her.

"Let's get started," he began. "There are a couple of ways of going about this. One way is to get you started today on giving us a semen sample, which we would freeze, and then do another sample 48 hours later and then another one 48 hours after that. The samples would all be frozen indefinitely and used when you wish to. This is your best bet because we don't know yet if you will need chemo or radiation, both of which will make you sterile.

"The alternative is to first do a semen analysis and see how many sperm you have and how they are doing. When we have those results, you can decide what to do in terms of sperm banking. If, and right now it's a big if, you don't need additional treatment for the cancer, you may have enough sperm from the other testicle to impregnate your wife normally. But that is making a leap of faith that you won't need additional treatment.

"My professional opinion is that the latter wastes time. If we get you started now, you can make a donation every 48 hours and therefore have more samples for future use. When you want to get pregnant, we can then inseminate your wife, which is a minor procedure. Not as much fun as the normal way, but we do play music and dim the lights."

Simon's head was once again reeling with all the information. Tara jumped in. "Just tell us what to do, Dr. Forester, please. It's been an awful day, and I just can't take anymore in. I need someone to tell us what to do." This time Simon agreed with her and nodded his head in agreement with his wife.

"Well, I would suggest that we get you started right away," the doctor responded. "The nurse will explain what needs to be done in terms of getting the first sample. You'll also need to get some blood drawn today or tomorrow to test for sexually transmitted infections and the like. The nurse will also talk to you about the costs involved in all of this. Ready?" And with that, he shook their hands and left the room. A middle-aged woman with red spiky hair came into the room within a few seconds. Simon and Tara did not look at each other while she briskly explained that Simon would need to masturbate into a cup, and that would be his first sample. She took them to a small room with a TV, a stack of DVDs, and some magazines. She told Tara that she could stay and help him if she wanted, but Tara just gasped and asked where the waiting room was. Simon entered the small room and closed the door. There was a small door set in the wall with a sign explaining that the sample cup should be placed on the other side of the door and a button pressed when the patient was finished. Simon could not believe this was happening to him and got down to business with a sense of resignation. When he finished, he joined Tara in the waiting room. This was his wife, but he had never felt more awkward in his life. The nurse invited them to a small office where she had some pamphlets for them. She quickly went over the costs of the sperm banking and storage. Simon couldn't help raising his eyebrows at the cost of all of this. No wonder the clinic was so plush. He felt guilty even thinking those thoughts and made a promise that he would never say anything about that to Tara. They left the clinic; it was almost 5 pm and the rest of the world looked normal. Would they ever be normal again?

Dr. Katz Explains

Sperm can be stored indefinitely in special tanks filled with liquid nitrogen. When a couple wants to get pregnant, samples are thawed and then placed into the uterus of the woman with a very thin tube. This is done at a time when she is ovulating and has the best chance of conceiving. An analysis of the sperm within the semen is performed routinely as part of the banking, storage, and insemination process, and the doctors will know if the man's sperm are behaving normally. A number of procedures can be done to maximize the number and health of the sperm so that the insemination has the best chance of success.

Sperm banking is to date the only tried and tested method of fertility preservation. Options for women are much more limited because eggs and ovarian tissue do not freeze well. A great deal of research is happening in this area of medicine, but at the present time, the only successful option for women is to stimulate the ovaries to produce many eggs, which are then mixed with sperm in the lab to create embryos . The embryos can be frozen and stored and later implanted into the woman's uterus. For women with cancer who need immediate treatment, the time needed to stimulate the ovaries to produce many eggs may delay treatment beyond a safe period. Futhermore, if the woman has to have her uterus removed, someone else will need to carry the pregnancy.

This entire process is expensive, and storage of sperm can run into the thousands of dollars over the years. Most fertility clinics have flexible financial plans to help couples do this. Most insurance plans do not cover fertility services.

The News Was Not Good

Simon had the surgery the following Wednesday morning. The intervening week had been terrible. They had to tell their parents and their closest friends, and Simon had to tell his colleagues at work. Tara asked her supervisor at the university to delay some of her research. All of this meant saying the same things over and over to different people many times during the next few days. Most people reacted with shock and did not know what to say. Simon and Tara quickly learned to recite the facts and to do so without their hearts being involved. Simon had also managed to make three separate donations at the fertility clinic, and he told himself that he had enough stored in the clinic to populate half the town.

The surgery itself was quite quick, and Simon went home later that day. His scrotum ached, and he was too afraid to feel down there. The urologist had talked to him about inserting a prosthetic testicle at a later date to make things look normal, but that could only be done after they knew whether he needed additional treatment. He had an appointment for the following week to hear the results from the pathologist and to learn whether radiation or chemotherapy would come next.

Tara had grown calmer over the past week. The night before the surgery, they had tried to make love, but it seemed to be a desperate act for both of them. After a few minutes they stopped and just held each other. She stayed at home with Simon as he recuperated over the next week and seemed to be almost her old self at times. Simon's office couriered over some files for him to work on at home, and he found the work to be a good distraction.

Exactly a week after his surgery, Simon and Tara were once again at the urologist's office. The news was not what they had hoped for: He was going to need radiation therapy and chemotherapy, but his prognosis was still good. The tumor was not large, but it had characteristics of two kinds of cancer, and so he needed dual therapy to give him the best chance of survival. He could feel Tara tense up. He grabbed her hand and squeezed it. He felt strangely calm and had a sense that it was going to be all right. But he knew that the next few months were going to be tough.

Five weeks later he started treatment. He had gone back to work a couple of days after hearing what the pathology showed, but he was distracted and had many appointments at the cancer center with different kinds of oncologists. In a way he was happy to begin treatment. His rationale was that the sooner he started, the sooner it would be over. His parents had been devastated with the news. His mother had taken to fussing over him as if he were a little boy. His father could barely bring himself to ask how Simon was feeling. Every time Simon said anything about the cancer or the treatments, tears would come to his dad's eyes, and he would walk away.

Take-Away Points

- Tell one or two good friends what has happened and let them tell everyone else. This limits your exposure to others' reactions and means you don't have to tell your story over and over.
- Discuss with your partner how to deal with your parents' responses. The two of you need to agree on how much they are involved in your day-to-day life.

Dr. Katz Explains

Having two kinds of cancer treatment can be challenging, as each has its own side effects, and the combination can be harsh. But Simon is a young man, an athlete, and he will recover. The time before treatment starts is often very difficult. Telling multiple people that you have cancer and seeing their reactions is draining. Sometimes you find yourself having to support these people when they hear the news instead of them supporting you. And parents will often revert to an earlier way of interacting with you and start treating you like a child again. You may not mind this, but it can cause problems if your partner doesn't like it!

Have You Had the Sex Talk?

Simon actually didn't mind the time he spent at the cancer center. That was strange and something he did not anticipate. He went every day for radiation, and beyond feeling embarrassed to have the whole team staring at his genitals, it really was not that bad. The chemotherapy treatments took a lot longer, but the treatment room was pleasant. Plus, if he went later in the evening, he could usually get a private room where he could watch DVDs or read. He had expected to feel nauseated by the treatment, but he was actually fine most of the time. He was very tired. Although he tried to eat healthy foods, he had some mouth ulcers that made eating fruits and vegetables difficult. It was easier to drink smoothies—luckily they had received a fancy blender as a wedding gift, and his mother took great pride in coming up with new combinations of flavors to stimulate his appetite.

About a week into treatment, a young nurse asked him if anyone had talked to him about sex. He almost laughed, but she had a really serious look on her face, and so he told her that his father had told him the basics when he was about 10 but since then he had figured it out on his own. The nurse started to laugh, which helped a bit. She explained to him that the chemotherapy in his body would be in his semen as well and he needed to wear a condom when having sex. Or not have sex at all. Simon couldn't help but smile ruefully when she said this. He was so exhausted and his mother was around so much that sex was the last thing on his mind these days. But he was grateful that she had explained this to him. Tara had been trying so hard to keep his spirits up. He could see the effort on her face when she joked and laughed in his presence, but he heard her crying in the bathroom almost every day, and she had delayed her graduate work for the whole semester. He didn't think this was a great idea, but she would not consider going back to her research. He could see the rationale for this—she was really having a hard time—but work had always been a distraction for him, and he thought it might be for her, too. But she was adamant that she would drive him to all his treatments. He insisted that she not stay while he had the chemotherapy. He liked the quiet of the treatment room and watching old war movies while the medication went in.

Dr. Katz Explains

Certain types of chemotherapy may be passed to one's sexual partner in semen (or vaginal fluids in women). You should use condoms if you plan to have sexual intercourse to protect your partner from the chemotherapy. Staff should always discuss this with patients before treatment is started, but this important piece of information may be missed. The patient can also forget it among all the other new information that has to be absorbed. Sometimes healthcare providers assume that someone having chemotherapy will not be having sex because he or she will feel too ill, but this assumption is often incorrect. Some healthcare providers also find it difficult to talk about sex with their patients and so may avoid the topic unless the patient asks a direct question about it. Or, they may assume that

Take-Away Points

- Always ask your healthcare providers if you are unsure about something. They may assume that you have read and understood all the information related to your treatment, when this may not be the case.
- You will probably need to use condoms for sex while having chemotherapy; if no one has talked to you about this, just ask.

the patient has read this information in one or more of the many books and pamphlets provided at various stages of the treatment process. Some patients find the amount of written information that they are given to be overwhelming and don't read anything, so it is important for healthcare providers to check if the patient has the correct information and has understood it.

Getting Back to Life

Six months later, Simon felt much better. He'd had his last chemotherapy treatment, and the radiation treatment was a distant memory. He was bald and had lost about 10 pounds off his already lean frame, but he was on the other side of the treatment phase and wanted to get back to his old life. Tara liked the way his head felt, hard and yet soft at the same time, and she secretly hoped he would shave his head from now on. When she told him this, Simon burst out laughing. But that night he looked at himself in the mirror and also liked what he saw. It reminded him a bit of the Olympic swim team. And it seemed to be attractive to his wife.

He went back to work part-time at first; he was really tired and found it hard to concentrate for more than a couple of hours. But each day he noticed a difference in his energy level, and his interest in work started to increase. He had always been competitive in everything he did, and now he set himself goals for each day. He had the occasional bad day when he couldn't meet his goal, but there were also lots of good days when he exceeded what he had set out to do. He even found himself thinking about sex more often. Even though Tara seemed scared to try, he wanted to, and one night she got a little drunk over dinner and agreed. It didn't last long—she was almost falling asleep, and it had been so long for him that it was over in just a few minutes. But it felt good, and he felt alive and normal. He added sex to his list of goals for every day and managed to meet that goal at first only once a week, and then more often. Tara was a bit irritated when she discovered this, but eventually she laughed about it. It was just such a Simon thing to do! And she had a deal for him, too. She had still not gone back to her graduate work, and she wanted to have a baby. She wasn't sure what he would say, but she was going to bring it up later that evening, maybe after dinner before either of them got involved with watching a TV show or Simon started doing some work. She had her arguments all prepared; she could be very persuasive if she wanted to be. But there would be no tears, just perfect logic and perhaps an attempt to play on his male pride. They'd been through so much this past year from the joy of their wedding to the shock of his diagnosis and the challenges of his treatment. Wanting a baby was in part a celebration, a confirmation of their hope for the future, and perhaps even some savings on the storage costs of all that semen. Tara had a plan!

CHAPTER 11

Sexuality and Terminal Illness

Just this once . . .

It may seem strange to think that people in the terminal stages of their cancer have sexual needs, but the desire for closeness and touch do not end when the end of life is near. In this chapter, readers will hear the story of Grant, a young man with leukemia. His girlfriend stays with him every hour that she can and tries her best to keep him comfortable. She is a little surprised when one day when his mother goes to the salon and he asks her to lie next to him in bed and take her clothes off.

From Grant's story you will learn
- How even at the end of life, people have the need for intimacy
- How some couples find compromise under difficult circumstances
- About the need for privacy when care is provided at home.

Grant's Story

Grant is only 22 years old and nearing the end of his life. He was diagnosed with an aggressive form of leukemia, acute myeloid leukemia (AML), just four and a half months ago. He has not had any luck in terms of his treatment. He had his first cycle of chemotherapy just two weeks after the diagnosis was made, and it did not lead to a remission of his cancer. He received another round of chemotherapy that the cancer also didn't respond to, and then a third. Each round of chemotherapy lasted about a month and made him feel terrible. He had to be really careful about avoiding people and crowds in case it exposed him to infection. The chemotherapy made him feel nauseated all the time, and sometimes he threw up for what seemed to be hours. Of course he had nothing in his stomach, so it was mostly dry heaves, which made his stomach muscles ache. After three cycles he told the doctors that he wanted to stop and just let whatever was going to happen, happen. His parents were devastated. They wanted him to continue fighting even though the doctors told him that it was likely of no use. The medical and nursing team were supporting Grant in his wish to spend the last weeks or months of his life with no treatment other than pain medication if needed and anything else that might help him be more comfortable.

Take-Away Points

- The decision to stop treatment is a difficult one.
- It is also one that may cause a great deal of distress to one's family, who may want the patient to continue with treatment at any and all cost to keep the person with them for as long as possible.

Dr. Katz Explains

Different kinds of leukemia exist, some more aggressive than others. AML is a cancer affecting the blood and bone marrow. The cancer affects immature blood cells that mature into red and white blood cells and platelets. AML is usually quite aggressive with rapid progression. Some people respond well to the chemotherapy during the induction phase of treatment. That is usually followed by consolidation therapy, which is given to maintain remission. But some people do not respond to the induction chemotherapy, and despite repeated cycles of chemotherapy, they do not go into remission. At that point, some may choose to not have any further treatment and let the disease take its course.

Mother Bird

Grant's girlfriend, Angie, was also very upset by his decision. They had started dating just three months before he was diagnosed, and she was terrified that he was going to die. She had seen him get so sick from the chemotherapy, but she also liked him a lot and hoped and prayed that he would be all right. She didn't have anyone to talk to about this. Her parents were not that keen on her dating him; she was 18 years old, and they thought he was too old for her. And then he got sick, and they thought she should get out of the relationship before she got hurt. So she didn't tell them anything about what was going on with him and also didn't tell them that she was skipping school most afternoons to spend time with him at home. He slept a lot of the time now, so she was able to keep up with her homework for school, and so far she had handed in all her assignments.

Grant's mom had been really nice to her. Her name was Barb, and she sometimes took off for an hour in the afternoon when Angie was at the house. Barb didn't want to leave Grant alone at home, and Angie was happy to help. It was also easier for her and Grant to talk when his mom wasn't around. His mom hovered over Grant, and no matter what he said, she still hovered. It was almost funny in a way, the way she constantly asked what he wanted and checked on him every few minutes. It reminded Angie of those birds that flitted around their nest when they had babies in there. But the reason that she was doing this wasn't funny, and Grant got really irritated with her sometimes. He said that he and Angie had no privacy, and he wasn't a little kid. That was true. But Angie liked knowing that his mom was around.

He had so much equipment in his room now; the oxygen canister that arrived just this week to help him breathe, the bell that he could ring if he needed anything, and of course the many bottles of pills with medication for pain and everything. Sometimes Angie was scared that something bad would happen when she was in the room with him and she wouldn't know what to do. He spent all his time in bed now. Once a week his dad helped him shower, but that exhausted him, so most days he just washed with a basin. He hardly ate anymore and was really thin. She bought some of the candies that she knew he really liked, but he hardly ate those, either. She mostly sat by his bed, and they watched TV together. Really, she watched and he dozed. She tried not to take it personally, but sometimes it hurt.

Dr. Katz Explains

All of this is very common when someone nears the final days of life. The person may sleep a lot and seem to be losing interest in the things that used to interest him or her. The person may not eat or drink much, and this can be difficult for those around the person to see. Food has such value in our lives, and bringing food to one you love when he or she is sick is a way that we show how much we care.

The hovering that Grant's mother is doing is also common. Like a mother bird takes care of her nestlings, so too do human mothers.

Take-Away Points

- As the end of life approaches, many people sleep more and seem to lose interest in what is going on around them.
- Visitors may need to wear a mask over their nose and mouth to protect the person from infection and should wash their hands well with soap and warm water before and after being in the room with the patient.
- Anyone with a cold should not be in the same room as the patient.

Constant checking is both reassurance that the person is okay and also a way of monitoring any changes.

When someone has this kind of leukemia, the cells in the blood that normally carry oxygen, the red blood cells, are crowded out by cancer cells. When these cells are at low levels, the person may be very tired and sleep a lot and may also need extra oxygen to prevent him from feeling like he is short of breath. The person also will have low levels of white blood cells, which help to fight infection. Therefore, he may get sick from exposure to groups of people and won't have the necessary defenses to fight off infection.

Waiting

Grant and Angie had not done anything sexually since they started dating. It was a decision that had caused some conflict for them. Angie wanted to wait until she was married to be with someone, and Grant didn't. He'd had girlfriends before Angie, and he was four years older than she was. But Angie stood her ground; she had strong religious views about this and was not prepared to compromise her beliefs. This was something she had been taught at home and at church, and she wanted to save herself for her husband. And anyway, they had only been dating for three months before he got sick. The months that he had been on chemotherapy he'd been too sick to really hassle her about this, and since he stopped treatment, he'd been too tired and weak. And she could see that he was getting weaker, although she didn't want to think what that meant.

If she really thought about it, she knew they would have probably broken up because of her desire to wait and his thinking that was dumb. So for the last three months since he got really sick, they didn't have to talk or fight about it, and it was easier that way. She could sit with him every day and stroke his hand and help his mom take care of him. He seemed to like having her around, and she felt like she was important in some way.

They also had no privacy anymore. Two days before, he'd had a nosebleed. Luckily it was when his mom was in his room changing the sheets. He'd moved to a chair, and boom—just like that the blood had come pouring out his nose.

Angie showed up just after it happened, and she felt sick to her stomach when she saw how much blood there was. It was all over the front of his T-shirt and was stuck to his upper lip; some had even dripped onto his chin.

His mom looked pretty freaked out about it too, and she started ordering Angie around the moment she walked into the room. Angie had to run to get a basin of water, and all she could find in the kitchen was a big salad bowl. She was scared that Barb would yell at her for bringing the wrong thing. But she didn't. It took them a long time to clean Grant up. He should have had a shower, but there was no way he could do that by himself, and there was no way he was going to allow his mom to see him naked. So they cleaned him up as best they could and helped him get into bed, which was clean and fresh from the new sheets. His mom called the nurse at the clinic, who said she had done the right thing. They also suggested that Grant could come in to have a blood transfusion, but he was just too wiped out to even think about it.

Dr. Katz Explains

Low levels of platelets, which help blood to clot, usually cause bruises, and some people get nosebleeds if they sneeze or blow their nose or just spontaneously. This can be very frightening for everyone, including the patients themselves. A transfusion of blood can temporarily provide platelets to help the blood clot. This may prevent another bleed but usually not for long.

In the Middle of It All

The nosebleed must have really scared Grant's mom, because that night she moved his bed into the family room downstairs. She said she was worried about something happening when she was in the kitchen. It wasn't really his bed that got moved, because he had a queen-size bed; she got Grant's dad to move a single bed from the spare room into the living room. The living room had a great view of the garden and the street beyond it, but Grant didn't seem to be interested in that.

He told Angie that he hated being down there. It was noisy and he didn't have any of his stuff around him anymore. Some of the furniture had to be moved down to the basement to make room for the bed, and he thought it was a lot of fuss for no good reason. But he was too tired to argue with his mom, and maybe it did make it easier for her. She was overweight, and he knew that going up and down the stairs a million times a day was hard for her. But now he really had no privacy. His mom was around all the time, and if someone came by to see her or bring food for the rest of the family, then he had to see them, too. Most of the people were friends of his parents. He really didn't want them to see him, and he didn't care to see them. There was a door to the living room, and he asked his mom to close it when someone was ringing the doorbell.

Take-Away Points

- If moving the sick person out of his or her bedroom seems to be the best option, try to find a room that has a door to minimize noise and give the person some privacy.
- Try to limit the times that visitors can come around; this will allow for some downtime for everyone.

Dr. Katz Explains

Having the sick person downstairs or in a central position in the house can make it much easier for caregivers. Going up and down stairs continually can be very tiring. But it does have the disadvantage of lessening any privacy for the person who is in the bed, and this can be a significant source of stress. Being in the middle of all the action can also be very tiring for the sick person, who will probably be disturbed when the phone rings or there is someone at the front door.

Just One Time

One afternoon in the same week that Grant had moved downstairs, Barb asked Angie if she would be okay for an hour alone with him. Barb needed to get her hair cut, and Angie had to inwardly admit that it was, in fact, true. Her roots were all gray, and her hair had completely lost its shape, but of course Angie didn't say anything like that out loud. She agreed to stay with Grant, but inside she was scared. What would she do if his nose started to bleed, or if something else happened? She wasn't sure what she would do or how she would act in an emergency. But she also knew it was a big deal that Barb had even asked her to do this. So she said yes.

Grant seemed to have been sleeping when she entered the living room. He had the oxygen tubing in his nose and there was a faint hissing sound in the room.

The blinds were closed and the room was a beige color without the sunshine coming in the windows. She sat down quietly next to him, trying not to disturb him. He had his MP3 player playing, and she thought he was asleep. She was really surprised when he spoke: "Is my mom out of the house yet? Is she?" Angie had heard the car backing out the drive, and she told him that she was gone and had said she'd be about an hour.

"Okay then, Angel" (that's what he called her). "Can you do something for me? Just one time. I want you to come and lie in the bed with me." Angie was not sure what to say. The bed was so small that she thought there wouldn't be any room for her. But his voice was pleading, and she didn't think about it for long. She tried to get him to move to the side of the bed but then got scared that he could fall off the other side, so she just lay on her side next to him.

"Angel, can you maybe take your clothes off? Just this once? I need to feel like I'm a guy and not some baby. I always wanted to see you like that and I thought we'd have time . . ." Just these few sentences took his breath away, and she could see his chest rising and falling rapidly under the sheets. She stood as still as a statue next to his bed, but her mind was racing. Why was he asking her to do this? He knew how she felt about this. But he sounded so desperate, and she wanted to make him happy. She slowly unbuttoned her shirt and pulled it over her head. Then she took off her jeans. Now she was standing in just her underwear and socks, and she felt stupid and scared and cold. She glanced at him. All she could see were his big brown eyes shining in the dim light. He was staring at her, and she didn't want to see him looking at her like that. She quickly pulled her bra over her head and then slipped her panties down and kicked off her socks. She lay down next to him, silently asking God to forgive her.

Dr. Katz Explains

Although this was very difficult for Angie, it shows clearly that even at the end of life, we are still essentially the person who we were before we got sick. Grant is doing something that most 22-year-old men want to do. He wants to see his girlfriend naked. Angie may have some issues in the future if she thinks that her actions on this day have compromised her faith, but she may also be comforted by knowing that she gave him a gift in his last days.

Thank You

Angie wasn't sure what she was supposed to do once she lay down next to him. She was scared that she was going to fall off the bed, and she was really scared that his mom would come back. The door to the living room was open, so she thought she would hear the car. She had locked the front door, so no one could just walk in. She lay next to him, holding her breath and hardly touching him. And then his arm moved toward her, and she took in a quick gasp of air. His hand rested on her tummy and he opened his fingers so that his hand was like a starfish. Her skin was all goose bumpy, and she didn't know what to do. He moved his hand from side to side. It felt light and heavy at the same time. She let him touch her skin, and she could feel his breathing grow faster. After a few minutes his hand stopped moving, and he whispered so softly that it was more like a breath. "Thank you, Angel. That was so good." And then he slept.

CHAPTER 12

Gay Men and Cancer

I have needs.

Michael and Jeff have been together for almost 20 years. Most of their friends are in committed relationships, and some of them have even married. But Michael and Jeff are the longest surviving couple in the group. They saw many friends die in the early years of the AIDS epidemic and have always been grateful that they were spared. But last year, Jeff was diagnosed with brain cancer. Since then, their sex life has essentially been over. Michael is happy that the love of his life is alive, but he misses their sex life and is having a difficult time dealing with the enforced abstinence that he has to live with now.

From Jeff and Michael's story you will learn

- How a change in personality in one partner affects the other
- About enforced abstinence and how it affects the partner.

Michael's Story

Michael and Jeff met in the summer of 1989 at a rally for AIDS funding. Those were desperate times, and yet there was an intensity to everything that happened, and that was intoxicating. They were both in their mid-thirties and settled in their careers, if not in their personal lives. There was so much to do in the fight against HIV/AIDS in those early years: They were fighting for healthcare services for their community, they were fighting the bureaucracy that didn't respond to what was happening, and they were fighting to keep themselves going when their friends were dying around them.

Every weekend there was one or more rallies, and both Michael and Jeff went to as many as they could. It felt good to be fighting and yelling against something instead of attending funerals and wakes. And at one of those rallies, they noticed each other and started talking. The attraction was instant. Now, 20 years later, they were fighting something again, but this time they were alone. The nightmare started about 15 months ago. Jeff had been complaining of headaches for a while, but of course he didn't do anything about it. Despite Michael's pushing every day, Jeff never made an appointment to see his physician. And one day he had a seizure at work. They called Michael from the hospital where the ambulance had taken him; Michael rushed over and then waited for what seemed like hours until someone came out and told him what was happening. Jeff had a tumor (they called it a "mass") in his frontal lobe. He was going to need more tests to find out exactly what kind of tumor it was, and then a treatment plan would be made. For a moment, Michael couldn't breathe and wasn't sure if his heart was still beating. But then he inhaled, and exhaled, and he knew that this was going to be the hardest fight of their lives.

Within days they had the diagnosis (it was an astrocytoma, a malignant kind of tumor), and Jeff was going to need treatment with a gamma knife, a special kind of radiation, as well as chemotherapy. Jeff was pretty out of it for those first few days. He had a difficult time taking in all the information that the doctors told them, and Michael had to repeat things to him over and over. Their friends rallied around as Michael knew they would; he made one phone call from the emergency room and within an hour had received more than 20 calls on his cell phone from friends offering help and support and love. While Jeff was in the hospital, some of their friends took turns walking his dog, Muffin, and there was always food in the fridge for Michael when he came home. Jeff was released five days after the seizure, and his treatment started the following week.

Dr. Katz Explains

Tumors in the brain aren't always cancerous, but in Jeff's case, it was an astrocytoma, which is malignant. Treatment of brain cancer is dependent on where and how large the tumor is. There are many treatments available, including surgery, different kinds of radiation, and also different kinds of chemotherapy. A delicate balance is required to eradicate the cancer and at the same time protect the brain against damage from the treatment itself.

The Trials of Treatment

Jeff's treatment was traumatic for them both. The gamma knife itself was not that bad, but he had to have metal screws inserted into the bones of his face and skull to hold a special cage over his head that was used to guide the radiation treatment. Jeff was horrified with this and wouldn't allow anyone to see him. He even tried to get Michael to stay at home and not come to the hospital, but there was no way that his partner of 20 years was going to stay away. Michael sat with him as they waited for the treatment to start. It was only at the last minute that he left Jeff with the nurses and radiation therapists. And he sat alone in the waiting room until someone came to tell him that the treatment was over and Jeff could go home.

Jeff slept a lot after the gamma knife treatment. Michael had been warned that this might happen, but he hadn't expected to find it so hard. He tried to entice Jeff to go for a short walk or to see friends or even to watch a movie with him. But Jeff seemed to have lost interest in everything around him. Michael hoped this was temporary, but the days slipped by. They'd been told that it might take months before they knew for sure that the cancer was gone, and Jeff was going to need tests to monitor his progress.

Michael had taken a leave from his job as an advertising executive in a firm he had helped to found 15 years before. His partners were good friends, and they had been so understanding and supportive when Jeff first got sick. But now he felt a little guilty being away from work; it wasn't like he was doing anything for Jeff. Jeff just stayed in bed most of the time. He ate if something was put in front of him, and he drank from the glass that Michael left next to the bed. But he did nothing of his own volition. If Michael didn't insist that he shower, he probably wouldn't even do that. But Michael wasn't sure that Jeff would be safe in the house if he was alone, so he stayed off work.

One day, Bradley, one of the other partners at the firm, called. Michael could hear how carefully he was choosing his words. One of their biggest accounts wanted Michael, and Michael only, to work on a new campaign for them. Bradley was apologetic, but that was what the client wanted, and he needed Michael to tell him what to do. Michael hesitated for only an instant and told Bradley that he would be back at work on Monday. He just needed a day or two to sort out some household help. In the meantime, he asked Bradley to send over copies of the work they had done for the client in the past.

Take-Away Points

- Supportive therapy such as occupational or physiotherapy can be useful in helping the patient regain lost function.
- If supportive therapy is not offered as part of treatment, you may have to ask for it on behalf of the patient.
- Consider what other life events may be influencing the patient's reaction to the diagnosis of cancer.

Dr. Katz Explains

Gamma knife is a special kind of radiation treatment that is targeted at the cancer cells in the brain. The radiation from the gamma knife prevents cancer cells from reproducing, so the effects of the treatment can take months to be seen. It is not uncommon for patients to feel tired after the gamma knife treatment. There is also a lot of emotion related to having cancer and the uncertainty of waiting to find out if the treatment has worked. This in itself can cause fatigue.

With brain cancer, the side effects related to the location of the cancer are sometimes the most significant factor. Jeff has a tumor in his frontal lobe, the area of the brain that is involved in personality as well as what are described as *executive functions* of the brain. These include decision making and rational thinking, as well as abstract thought and planning. Jeff's behavior following his diagnosis and treatment suggest some impact on his frontal lobe, either from the tumor itself or from swelling in the area after the radiation from the gamma knife.

However, as a gay man who has survived the HIV/AIDS epidemic without becoming infected, Jeff may be angry that after all he did to protect himself from that deadly infection, he now has a different deadly disease. This anger may manifest as depression, withdrawal, or ineffective coping.

Where Did He Go?

A few weeks after the gamma knife treatment, Jeff started chemotherapy. He was taking a cocktail of different drugs, and he was sick most of the time. A group of their friends had formed themselves into a team to care for Jeff. Some of them worked nights and were able to take him to the hospital for his treatments during the day. Someone always waited at the house until Michael came home. He'd gone back to work and felt guilty that he wasn't there for Jeff during the day. But the truth was that he found it really difficult to see Jeff so sick. Evenings and weekends were bad enough. There were times when he found himself staring at this man whom he had loved for 20 years and wondering, where did he go? Where was the Jeff that he had fallen in love with and made a life with?

The man who lived with him now was like a hologram of the vibrant, handsome man he used to be. Jeff had lost almost all his hair, about 45 pounds, and the essence of who he once was. The man who was left didn't talk, didn't express emotion, and mostly just sat where he was left. The nurses had told him that the chemotherapy was going to be rough, and he had expected some nausea and vomiting. He knew intellectually that Jeff would lose his hair and some weight, but what he didn't expect was that Jeff was going to look like someone with AIDS. There! He had thought it! Jeff looked like he had AIDS. This realization overwhelmed Michael and his eyes filled with tears. In a way it also helped him—a wave of sympathy swept over him. This was something he could deal with! He knew what to do. Twenty years ago he had cared for so many friends with that horrible disease, and he could do it again.

Dr. Katz Explains

Take-Away Points

It is often difficult to anticipate the changes that may occur when someone is going through treatment. Not everyone responds in the same way, but weight loss and hair loss are quite common during chemotherapy. Jeff is also experiencing some cognitive and emotional changes, most likely because of where the tumor is in his brain,

- Consider previous experiences of loss when trying to understand reactions to a life-threatening illness.
- Everyone experiences illness in his or her own unique way; there is no right or wrong way to behave.

and this in many ways is much more difficult to watch and deal with. Many people with brain cancer undergo personality changes, and for those who love them, it may feel like they are not the same person anymore.

For gay men who lived through the HIV/AIDS epidemic, the weight loss associated with cancer and treatment may subconsciously be associated with the weight loss of those with advanced AIDS. Although Michael intellectually recognizes that Jeff only looks like he has AIDS, there may be a powerful internal struggle with this realization that potentially can draw him closer to his partner or perhaps disengage from him. Jeff's altered appearance may remind both of them of the multitude of losses they experienced during the height of the HIV/AIDS epidemic when so many died.

Other Changes

Jeff finished his chemotherapy and, over the next few weeks, started to gain weight and look more like his old self. The group of friends looking after him while Michael was at work had all shaved their heads as a sign of support (not Michael, however), and as the weeks went by, their hair started to grow back and they called themselves the "Easter Chicks." Gradually Jeff gained strength and was able to look after himself more and more. But he wasn't the same as he used to be, and their relationship was different, too. It had been some months since they had shared a bed. Although it made sense in the beginning when Jeff was so sick, for some reason they remained in their separate bedrooms.

Michael wasn't sure what was going on, but things felt really different. He tried not to think about it and told all their friends how happy he was to have the old Jeff back. But that wasn't quite the whole truth. Jeff was different; he was quieter and hardly ever laughed the way he used to. He seemed content just to sit in the house, petting Muffin and watching TV. They hadn't kissed or shown any other kind of physical affection toward each other since he got sick. Michael wasn't sure that this was normal, but then again, what was normal? Their world had shifted, and he had a sinking feeling that nothing was going to be the way it was before.

One day their friend Roger was over for a drink. He and Jeff had been lovers many years ago, and Roger was never one to hold anything back. He cornered Michael in the kitchen when he went to get more ice and limes for their drinks. "Hey, old friend," he began. "Methinks things are not what they seem." Michael looked at him, taking his time to formulate a response. Roger was a good friend, but he had a nasty habit of asking about things that were better left unspoken. "What do you mean?" he asked, trying to keep his voice light. "You and Jeff is what I mean," replied Roger, his face serious and his tone measured. "I think there's something else going on, or not going on, if you get my meaning." Michael definitely "got his meaning." It had been months since he and Jeff had slept in the same bed, but he didn't want to talk to Roger about this. He brushed him off as best he could and went back out to the deck, the limes and ice forgotten.

Even though he didn't want to, he thought about Roger's words a lot over the next few days. He knew that he felt differently toward Jeff; he just didn't know how or why. One night he decided to see what would happen if he tried to touch Jeff. After dinner he put his arms around the man he had loved for two decades. And nothing happened. His heart didn't skip a beat, and the rest of his body didn't react either. Jeff shook off his arms and went back to watching an episode of some detective show. Michael was shocked at both his and Jeff's responses. What did this mean? He knew in his heart that he loved Jeff, but he no longer wanted him in a physical way. And Jeff seemed to not want any kind of physical touch either. What now?

Dr. Katz Explains

Take-Away Points

- Some couples do grow apart after cancer and its treatments.
- There is no right or wrong way to deal with changes in sexual attraction.

There are many reasons why Jeff rebuffed Michael and why Michael felt little when he touched his partner of 20 years. Jeff seems to have changed, and Michael has changed too. The sexual spark that existed in their relationship seems to be missing. Can it be brought back? Does either of them want it back? Sometimes the partners themselves may not notice that things have changed, and it takes an outsider to notice and point it out. Or, the knowledge that something has changed may be so painful that one or both partners prefer to not deal with it.

That sexual spark can be a very fragile entity; many factors affect it. Michael has seen physical and personality changes in his partner. He has had to provide daily care for him when he was sick and also now as he recovers. All of these may affect his attraction to his partner. And Jeff may be suffering the effects of the cancer and its treatments, all of which affect his sexual interest. And he may feel differently about Michael in the light of everything he has gone through.

What Am I Going to Do?

The weeks and months went by with things no different in Michael and Jeff's life. Jeff had not been able to go back to his job as the manager of a popular downtown restaurant and bar. He stayed at home most days watching TV. Michael was still very busy at work with new projects and campaigns holding his attention. He knew that he was using work as an excuse for not dealing with things at home, but it was just easier this way. He and Jeff were now housemates. Jeff kept himself busy caring for their dog, and he had many friends who came by often and took him out for lunch or coffee. Roger was one of his most faithful friends; he visited almost every other day. If Michael knew he was at the house, he tried to keep away. Roger was too observant and too forthright. He would ask questions, and Michael didn't want to think about the answers. He was Jeff's friend first and foremost. In a way, Michael was a bit scared of him and his loyalty to Jeff.

One evening Michael came home and Roger was there. Jeff was taking a nap in his favorite chair on the deck, and Michael couldn't avoid Roger when he confronted him in the kitchen. "So Mike," he began. "How are you doing, really?" Michael mumbled that he was doing just fine. He tried to busy himself with opening a bottle of wine and was disappointed to find that the bottle of New Zealand Sauvignon Blanc in the fridge had a screw cap; no need to search for a corkscrew or occupy himself with the ritual of getting the cork out. "It must be difficult for you, seeing Jeff this way." Michael was irritated with Roger's persistence. Not only was he aggressive in his protection of Jeff, but he was also a child psychologist and knew how to ask the hard questions. Michael was getting by as best he could. He didn't want anyone getting under his skin now or ever. But Roger just kept on asking questions, and suddenly Michael found himself pouring his heart out to Roger.

He told him that they were living like college housemates and that it was slowly killing him. He described how lonely he felt and how he missed the old Jeff with his sexy smile and ready laughter. Roger leaned against the kitchen table and listened. His eyes were warm and locked onto Michael's face as he spoke. He didn't say much, just nodded and allowed Michael to continue. Michael talked about still loving Jeff but no longer being in love. And when Roger asked about sex, he just laughed with a hollow sound. "I wasn't kidding about the housemate part," he replied. "That's all gone, and I don't know what I'm going to do. I have needs, you know, but I can't do anything about them. I never thought I'd be celibate at this stage of my life. I'm 55 years old and I'm living like an 80-year-old!" Roger reached out and put his hand on Michael's shoulder. "You need to deal with this, Michael. It's not going to go away. How about I set you up with a counselor at the clinic where I work. There are some good people there, and they're gay-friendly. I'll speak to someone tomorrow and get you in.

No arguments now; you know you need to do this." It was now Michael's turn to nod. He picked up the bottle of wine and three glasses and went out to the deck to wake Jeff.

Dr. Katz Explains

Take-Away Point
• Be open to opportunity. Help comes in different ways and often at times when you need it most.

Michael needs help, and sometimes help comes in an unexpected way or from an unexpected source. When he opened up to Roger, he had reached a point where in a way he was asking for help. He was unhappy with how things were going in his relationship. He felt disconnected from Jeff and tied to him at the same time. And he was experiencing sexual frustration and didn't know what to do about it. Roger offered professional help and didn't try to fix it himself. Even though Michael doesn't think of Roger as his friend, Roger has proved to be a better friend than many others.

I Need Help

The next day Roger called Michael at his office and told him that he had managed to get him an appointment with one of the counselors for 5 pm that day. Michael was a little surprised but also grateful. He called Jeff at home and told him he would be home later than usual. Jeff seemed his usual self and thanked Michael for telling him, and that was the end of the conversation. Michael just shook his head. In the past, Jeff might have pouted or moaned that Michael was not coming home at his regular time, but now he just accepted it as if he didn't care.

Michael left work and drove the short distance to the clinic where Roger worked as a psychologist. He had never been to see a counselor before, and he really didn't know what to expect. The clinic was in a nondescript building with a small courtyard facing the street. There was a parking lot across the street, and Michael recognized Roger's car parked there. The waiting room at the clinic was full; children played with toys in one corner, and their parents sat in worn chairs watching them. The noise level was high as the kids shouted and laughed. Michael's first instinct was to leave. What was he doing here? He stood at the reception desk while a young woman, presumably the receptionist, spoke on the phone. She nodded at Michael and held up one hand, indicating that she was busy but would get to him in a moment. The moment became minutes as she continued her phone conversation. Michael grew increasingly irritated and was just about to leave when he heard a familiar voice. "Hey, Mike!" It was Roger, and he knew he was trapped. "Come on through to my office, and I'll introduce you to the counselor. Just ignore Chatty Cathy over there—she's the world's worst receptionist, but she's all we can afford!" Michael was happy to leave the chaos and noise of the waiting room. He followed Roger into a narrow hallway. "I know it doesn't look like much," Roger explained as they walked down the hallway. "But we do good work here. There are fancier places, but the people here are dedicated, and more than that, they're good at what they do. Hey, I work here!" Michael smiled at Roger's self-confidence and followed him into a cramped office. He was not sure if he should sit, and Roger had disappeared. He returned within seconds with a woman in tow. "Michael, this is Joyce, the counselor I've arranged for you to see. She's small but mighty, and I think you two are going to get along just fine."

Michael was not sure why he felt so surprised. Roger had never said that the counselor was a woman, but Michael had just assumed that a gay-friendly counselor as promised would be a man, and a gay man at that! Instead he found himself shaking the hand of a short woman with cropped black hair. She had a warm smile and a firm handshake. Within a few seconds, she had extricated him from Roger's small office and taken him to a larger room with a couple of sofas and a large potted tree.

Joyce wasted no time. "What can I do for you, Michael?" she asked as she sat down. Michael took a deep breath. "I need help," he began, and as he said it he knew that it was true. "It's a long story . . . ." Joyce nodded her head and fixed her eyes on him. And he told her his story. He talked about loving Jeff and feeling imprisoned by that love. He talked about the bonds of 20 years and the frustration of living in a celibate relationship. Even to his ears he realized that his story sounded confused. He loved Jeff and yet was frustrated with the lack of physical contact between them. He didn't want to leave the relationship and yet he couldn't see himself remaining celibate for the rest of his life. Joyce asked some simple questions: Where was he finding sexual release? Had he thought about finding someone for an uncomplicated sexual relationship on the side? Michael was clear in his responses to her questions. Yes, he masturbated regularly, but that really didn't provide him with what he needed. And no, he was not prepared to look for sex outside the relationship. What a mess this all was! And how could anyone help?

Dr. Katz Explains

Take-Away Points

- The essence of a problem often becomes clearer when you talk about it out loud.
- What may seem like confusion to you may be much simpler in the eyes of a trained professional.

What sounds like a mass of contradictions is actually quite simple. Michael is missing the intimacy of a sexual relationship with someone he loves. Intimacy means the heart-to-heart connectedness that we strive for in our primary relationships. Michael is missing that special connection with his partner of 20 years. Masturbation could provide some temporary relief from sexual frustration, but it was not the same as a sexual relationship with someone that you love and who loves you back. Going outside the relationship for sexual gratification is not something that he wants to do, as he sees this as a betrayal of his relationship.

For a gay man in his 50s, finding someone else may be very difficult. Gay communities are often harsh in their rejection of older men (even in their 50s!), and the HIV/AIDS epidemic in many cities decimated men of Michael's generation. Michael will likely face quite a challenge finding someone in the gay community, even if he wanted to. This particular form of ageism may be somewhat unique to the gay community, but the fear of not being able to find love is universal for many who lose their partner.

Michael has been forced by a set of circumstances to be sexually abstinent. This is very different than the periods of abstinence that many people have before or between relationships. It is different because Michael does not see himself as having any choices—or rather he doesn't have a choice that he is willing to make. He wants to stay in his relationship but is having problems accepting what that means.

Telling It Like It Is

Michael listened to Joyce as she pointed out the key points as she saw them. Michael deserved praise for wanting to stick it out, for not wanting to go outside the relationship for sex. But she also wanted to know why he had given up after just one try at touching Jeff. This question stunned Michael; he had given up after only one attempt! That was not like him at all. Why had he given up so quickly? Was there more going on than he was willing to admit?

Joyce listened as he tried to work out the whys and whats of his recent history with Jeff. He admitted that Jeff's appearance after his treatment had been an issue for him. His resemblance to someone with AIDS had been shocking to Michael and may have played a role in his change of feelings. He also realized as he talked that he was afraid of losing Jeff, but at the same time he was having difficulty accepting this new Jeff who had emerged after treatment. And he was afraid of what would happen if this was really all that their relationship was going to be.

Michael eventually fell silent. There was so much more to this than he had thought. Joyce let him sit there for a few minutes and then she spoke. She told him that she was going to ask him to bring Jeff to another appointment with her. Michael opened his mouth to object or make an excuse, but Joyce stopped him. "I'm going to tell it like it is, Michael. This is not just your problem. Jeff has a voice, too. Or at least I hope to hear his voice. You need to bring him with you next time. This is something that the two of you need to deal with. While he's with you, it's his problem, too." Michael knew she was right. But how was he going to get Jeff to come with him to an appointment?

Dr. Katz Explains

Michael in his own way has had much to get used to since Jeff's diagnosis and treatment. It may sound selfish (and many partners of people with cancer feel a great deal of guilt about taking their feelings, wants, and desires into consideration), but the partner also experiences many changes in the face of cancer. It is very difficult to see someone suffer. It is also difficult to live with the aftermath, particularly where there has been a change in the appearance or personality of the other person.

A diagnosis of cancer is life threatening, and many people start the mourning process in anticipation. There is even a term for this: anticipatory grieving. Either the patient or the partner, or both, can begin this process. It often is manifested as withdrawal and distancing as one or the other—or both—prepare for life without the person with cancer. It may seem counterintuitive, to start mourning when the person is still there, but it is an unconscious protective mechanism, in part, and not a rational process.

A brain tumor may precipitate a different kind of mourning: the loss of the person who used to be. It can take a while for the partner to learn to love the new person who has made an appearance after the cancer. The person with cancer also may not feel like his or her old self and may have to make similar alterations to the way he or she thinks and feels. It's a two-way street with the potential for bumps and potholes along the way.

It's About Us

When Michael walked into the house a while later, Jeff was alone in the living room, the TV on and Muffin lying on his lap. Instead of going straight to the kitchen, Michael sat down next to him on the sofa. Jeff seemed a little surprised by this and sat there, as still as a statue. "Jeff, I need to talk to you about something," Michael said. "It's about us. I don't know where to start, but I saw a counselor today, about us. Well, about me, really. But she said it's about us, and she wants me to bring you to my next appointment." He'd said all that in one breath, and now Michael drew in a deep breath, waiting for Jeff to respond. "Okay" was all he got. But it was better than "no" or even "why." After 20 years, there was still much to learn. Jeff was different, and that meant that Michael was going to need to do things differently, too. It was a start.

PART THREE

Seeking Help

In this section, you'll learn about useful resources and strategies to get you on the road to sexual recovery. You'll also learn what happens to the partner of a man with cancer and how his cancer affected her and their relationship.

CHAPTER 13

The Partner of a Patient With Cancer

What happens to one partner when the other gets cancer?

When one member of a couple is affected by cancer, the partner suffers, too. This chapter will detail some specific sexual issues that can affect the partner. This chapter tells the story of George, a middle-aged man with prostate cancer. He is very concerned and frustrated about what has happened to his sex life, and he is taking this out on his wife, Joyce. He is demanding of her and even goes as far as suggesting that she needs to find someone else.

From George and Joyce's story, you will learn

- How some men have doubts about their masculinity after cancer treatment
- How not to deal with these issues.

George's Story

George was diagnosed with and treated for prostate cancer almost three years ago. His diagnosis came as a shock to him, and he was insistent that he have the surgery immediately. His wife, Joyce, went along with his decision. She'd learned over the 37 years of their marriage that when he made up his mind, that was it and there was no changing it. George didn't seek any help from her after he learned the news from the urologist to whom he had been referred. He didn't talk to his family doctor, who had been monitoring his prostate-specific antigen

(PSA) level, nor did he talk to his brother, who had been treated for the same cancer five years before.

His brother, Norman, was shocked to hear that George was having the surgery only three weeks after he was diagnosed. Norman was very active in a prostate cancer support group in the city where they both lived. When he had been diagnosed, he spent almost three months researching and then exploring his treatment options. Like George, his cancer was of the low-risk variety, and he had wanted to make sure that he did the right thing. He found out about the support group in his city and started going to the monthly meetings. The support group played an important part in helping him to decide on a treatment, and he maintained contact with them over the years. But George did what George always did—he decided on something without talking to anyone, including his wife, and that was that.

Take-Away Points

- Take your time in making a treatment decision; there is usually no need to rush.
- Attending a prostate cancer support group can be helpful, as you will meet other men who have been through the decision-making process.
- The decision is often difficult to make with all the factors that have to be weighed against each other.

Dr. Katz Explains

Depending on the stage and grade of the cancer found in the prostate, many men have options for treatment. Some men may be able to delay treatment by being closely monitored on a regular basis with PSA tests and repeated biopsies. This is called *active surveillance* and may be a good choice for men with low-risk, low-volume disease who are interested in delaying or deferring treatment. The most common treatment for prostate cancer is surgical removal of the prostate. This may be done through an incision in the abdomen or by laparoscopic technique with or without robotic assistance. Another option is radiation therapy, either via external beam or the placement of radioactive seeds directly into the prostate. Research suggests that men choose their treatment based on what kind of specialist they see; those who see a surgeon are more likely to have surgery, and those who see a radiation oncologist have radiation therapy.

In today's world, prostate cancer usually is diagnosed after a biopsy is performed because the PSA level is raised. Most of these cancers are diagnosed in the early stages with low or intermediate grades, allowing for the man to choose what treatment he wants. Both surgery and radiation are equally effective in treating this kind of prostate cancer, and men are encouraged to decide on their treatment based on a detailed discussion of the risks and benefits of each. Treatment for prostate cancer will affect quality of life, and each man will have his own opinion about what that will mean for him. The important thing is to take some time in making that decision and to find help in weighing the pros and cons of each kind of treatment.

Just Get It Out

George called the urologist two days after he received the diagnosis. He asked for a surgery date as soon as possible and told the doctor to just get it out. Three weeks later he had the surgery. His brother was shocked at his actions. George had seen an older urologist who was known in the prostate support group as someone who did not perform the newest surgical techniques, so George's surgery was not nerve-sparing, which is the usual way to do the surgery. Following the surgery, George had a lot of incontinence, and even three years later he still needed to wear a pad every day. He was frustrated and angry and took a lot of this out on his wife. He was also really bothered by the fact that he could no longer have erections. He didn't like to talk about it, but Joyce knew how depressed it made him. He had tried to find a solution to this, but the urologist had told him that once the nerves were gone, that was it. But from his perspective, the important thing was to cure the cancer. He suggested that George try the vacuum pump or injections, but George didn't want to use either.

Dr. Katz Explains

Wanting to do something about the cancer is a normal and expected reaction. Many men just want to have the prostate taken out, thinking that this is the end of their problems. If they then have ongoing incontinence, they often

Take-Away Points

- The type of treatment often dictates the kind of side effects you may experience.
- Treatments are available for the side effects, but their success is variable.

experience a significant decrease in quality of life. Some men with incontinence are reluctant to leave their home for fear of having an accident and become socially isolated. Erectile difficulties are common after surgical removal of the prostate, as you have read earlier, and if the nerves weren't spared during the surgery, almost all men will be unable to have erections, and the oral medications (sildenafil, tadalafil, vardenafil) will not be effective.

I Can't Stand Needles

Over the years following his surgery, George grew more and more despondent about the sexual side effects of his surgery. He was angry a lot of the time and took it out on Joyce. He had always had a bit of a temper, and she had learned how to deal with this over the many years of their marriage. But this was different. They were arguing almost every day, about the smallest of things, and there were times when she wondered if she should leave him, not forever but just to teach him a lesson. But she couldn't. She believed that you were married for life, for better or for worse, and she would stand by him even through the most difficult of times.

She begged George to consider using the injections, but he told her he couldn't stand the thought of putting a needle into his penis. She offered to do it for him, and this gave him pause for thought. She had talked to a woman that Norman had introduced her to. She didn't tell George about this; he would have been really angry had he known. This woman had told Joyce that after the first couple of tries with the needle, she had taken over this task because her husband hated injecting himself. She just shrugged her shoulders when Joyce asked her how she felt about this and if she was okay giving him the injections. Joyce knew what that shrug meant; sometimes you just have to do what you have to do to keep the peace. But George wouldn't hear of it, and once again, that was that.

Joyce wanted to do whatever she could for her husband. She could see how unhappy he was, and he was making her unhappy, too. He didn't want to do anything anymore. They used to have an active social life and had looked forward to traveling in their retirement. Since his surgery, their world had shrunk, and neither of them was happy. But George didn't seem to want to do anything about fixing this unhappiness. He seemed just fine about being angry and frustrated.

Dr. Katz Explains

Some people just don't like needles, and not much can be done about that. Even though the needle used for injecting the penis is the same size as the one that millions of diabetics use every day, the thought of putting any needle into the penis is too much for many men, and perhaps also their partners. It is actually a fairly simple procedure that can be easily taught and learned, but it is not so much about the technique but rather the attitude toward the needles themselves.

The changes in George and Joyce's relationship are more concerning. George is obviously upset about what has happened and is taking out his frustration on his wife. Joyce has even thought of leaving him, an indication of how unhappy she is. George seems to be unable or unwilling to accept any help from his wife; this is sad but not uncommon. Many men think that they have to fix everything, and if they can't, then it remains broken.

Introducing Bill

Over the past three months, George has become friendly with a man named Bill who lives in the same complex as the couple. The two men met at the mailboxes and started talking. In the past, George had always had a wide circle of friends, men with whom he played golf or cards. But since his surgery, his social life has really shrunk, and he hardly saw any of his old friends anymore. When Joyce encouraged him to contact some of these men, he snapped at her that he couldn't do the same things anymore because of the incontinence, and the subject was closed. Once again, that was that.

But now he had a new friend, one who didn't know him from the past and someone who George thought wouldn't judge him. Bill was about the same age as George, both in their mid-60s, and although they didn't have all that much in common, Bill was a nice sort of guy. He told George that his wife had died of some sort of cancer a year before he moved to the retirement complex. Bill hadn't wanted to stay in their home, and he thought he might meet new people if he moved to a place where there were people his own age.

George invited him over for a drink one weekend evening. Joyce was happy to see her husband had made a new friend, and she was gracious when Bill came around. The following week, George invited his new friend for coffee on two separate occasions. He didn't tell Joyce either time. She walked into their condo both days after running errands to find them sitting on the deck, talking. They seemed to get along well enough, although Joyce found him to be very quiet with little to say to her. But what was important was that George liked him, and she was grateful that he finally seemed to be coming around.

Dr. Katz Explains

Some men struggle with their identity after surgery for prostate cancer. This is more likely to occur if they think that they are less of a man as a result of the changes brought on by incontinence and especially inability to have an erection. They may stop seeing their friends and avoid social contact with those who knew them before. They wrongly assume that their friends know about their problems and think less of them because of this. This is an erroneous assumption, but as you have read before in this book, attitudes and beliefs are strong influences on behavior and often are not based in fact.

Reciprocity

Over the weeks, Bill seemed to be around more and more. At first it was for coffee or a drink on the weekend. But he seemed to linger more and more when he was over, and Joyce felt obliged to offer him dinner. George seemed pleased when she did this. Soon, Bill was having dinner with them two or three times a week. He seemed so thankful for their hospitality and would bring flowers or chocolates as a thank-you gift for the meal. On the weekends he would bring beer, and once a bottle of wine for Joyce. After three months in which he ate increasingly more of his meals at their condo, he invited them out for dinner as a thank-you. He wanted to reciprocate their hospitality, he explained, but he was a lousy cook and didn't want to punish them with his efforts in the kitchen. So he asked them to join him at a restaurant nearby.

Joyce was not thrilled about this; Bill was George's friend. While he was not offensive in any way, she did not really care for the man but tolerated him for George's sake. She and George arrived at the restaurant a few minutes late. George was wearing jeans and a sweater, and they had a fight about this that made them late. She wanted him to put on a shirt and jacket, but he refused. When they got to the restaurant, they had barely sat down with Bill when George got up and excused himself. He said that he had forgotten something and left the table before they could say anything. Joyce and Bill sat in awkward silence. Bill ordered a beer, and Joyce felt obliged to have a glass of wine with him. The minutes ticked by very slowly. Bill didn't talk much to her, and she kept looking at her watch. Where on earth was George? After about 20 minutes she excused herself and asked to use the restaurant phone. She was worried about her husband and feared that perhaps he was ill. His behavior was strange even for him!

She was very surprised when George answered the phone as if nothing was wrong. "Where are you? Are you okay? I'm worried about you. You just left, and I'm sitting here with Bill waiting for you." George was vague in his reply, suggesting that nothing was wrong, he was fine, but she should go ahead and have dinner with Bill, and he would see them later at the condo. This was a very strange response, thought Joyce, and she returned to the table. She told Bill that she had to leave, that George was not coming back and she was worried about him. Bill left some money on the table and they drove back in silence. Joyce was so embarrassed. When they reached the condo, she knocked on the door loudly. George came to the door, still dressed in his jeans and sweater. He smiled at Joyce and Bill and invited Bill to come in and have a cup of coffee. This was the last straw for Joyce—she turned to face Bill and told him that it was time for him to go home and that there would be no coffee for him that night. She looked at her husband of 37 years and asked him exactly what was going on. She'd had enough and wanted to know the truth.

George at first denied there was anything wrong. In his typical fashion he told her she was making things up, and she could tell that once again he was picking a fight. But this time she was determined to sort out his strange behavior, and she would not give in. After a few minutes, George told her his plan. He realized that he could no longer satisfy her, that he was not a whole man anymore, and that if she left him—and he wouldn't blame her if she did—then he thought he would help her to find someone else. He thought Bill would make a fine replacement and therefore had encouraged Bill to spend time with her. Nothing was wrong with his health that night when he left the restaurant; he just wanted them to spend some time alone and get to know each other better without him there. Joyce was speechless.

Dr. Katz Explains

George had devised a plan that was extraordinarily inappropriate, although at the same time so generous. He was trying to help his wife replace him! He had not talked to her about the need to replace him and was so misguided in his actions that it was almost comical. But the reasons for his actions are not comical at all. George is a man who has lost his masculine identity as a result of the side effects of treatment. Although his response of trying to fix his wife up with another man was inappropriate, it is a reflection of how bad he feels about himself. In a convoluted way, George was actually being very generous, but of course it may be difficult for Joyce to see this.

How Could You?

The only words to come out of Joyce's mouth were garbled. She was stunned at his behavior that night, and now that she understood what his plan was, she was stunned at his behavior leading up to this. "How could you even think that I wanted to replace you?" she asked her husband. "Why would you even think that?" George, for once, didn't try to bully her about her opinion. He actually looked a little sheepish, while at the same time a bit relieved with her angry response to his plan. "I cannot believe how stupid you can be, George. Even for you, this pretty much takes the cake. I am so angry right now that I am not sure I can talk to you. That may have to wait until tomorrow. But believe me, there *will* be a tomorrow, and we are going to talk this out. Good night." She left the room, entered the bathroom, and slammed the door. He had some explaining to do. They would talk tomorrow.

CHAPTER 14

Strategies to Ease the Tension

Couples can try some useful strategies to help them talk to each other and start the healing process. This chapter will address these strategies and provide couples and individuals with some of the words to use when discussing this sensitive topic with their sexual partner.

Superman?

One of the greatest myths in society suggests that all men are sexual machines. The expectation is that men can have sex on demand, at any time, in any place, no matter what his feelings or emotions are. This is often depicted in cartoons as men having a single on-off button—simple to use, and we all know what happens when the switch is in the "on" position. This myth is, in part, perpetuated by the introduction of pills like Viagra® (Pfizer Inc.). The inference is that if a man can have an erection, then everything is okay. Women, on the other hand, are shown as being extremely complex with many dials and switches. Women are expected to be complicated in their sexual responses and actions.

Talk, Talk, Talk

This chapter focuses on communication, an important part of everyday life and an essential part of a healthy relationship. Here's another myth: Men don't talk about their feelings and certainly don't want to talk about sex. Well, the last part may be partially true. It's not always easy to talk in a meaningful way about sex. We can joke about it, and many of us outright lie about it or just pretend. But really talking about it, from the heart, is more difficult for some of us.

Why is it so difficult to talk about sex? It seems to be the topic of many talk shows, and men's magazines (and some women's magazines, too) are full of articles about how to have more sex, how to last longer, and how to drive your partner wild. Music videos show people simulating having sex in cars, on rooftops, and so on, but is this real, or just some setup that ends up making many of us feel inadequate? Real discussions are not that simple. We don't see or hear meaningful discussions about sex, so we sometimes have difficulty talking about it in a meaningful way.

How did you learn about sex? Most of us learned about it from older siblings, friends at school, and "dirty" magazines that we found in our father's bedroom or that our friends brought to school. Young men today learn about sex on the Internet by watching porn sites. None of this is realistic. Most of our parents didn't talk to us in a meaningful way about healthy sexuality. You may have been warned about "being careful" and "not getting a girl into trouble" or how "nice girls don't or won't." None of these messages were about sexual pleasure and sexual health. Many men have grown up with negative messages about masturbation. These include beliefs that it is bad or wrong, second best to "real" sex, and many men carry guilty feelings about it throughout their lives. Masturbation is healthy and normal and serves many purposes, such as learning about what feels good, relief of tension, and relaxation.

All these factors influence how we think and talk about sex. And they influence your partner, too. Your healthcare providers are under the same influences, and this may be why they don't talk to you about sexual changes during and after cancer treatment. Most physicians and nurses only receive a couple of hours of education about human sexuality, so they often do not know how to talk about it to their patients.

But perhaps the biggest barrier to talking about sex is that we are afraid. What if we say the wrong thing and upset our partner? What if we say a word and she laughs? What if something we say hurts or offends our partner? Will we be rejected or made to feel like a fool for expressing our innermost feelings or fears? How do we talk about it?

Here are some suggestions to help you and your partner talk about sex (and love and passion and pain).

Find the time.

Just like any other important discussion you've ever had, you need to set aside time to talk about sex. This is not a conversation you should have while rushing to get to work. You probably find the time to plan a vacation, right? So find the time to talk about this important part of your relationship. Any problems you may be having did not start overnight, and they are not going to be solved overnight, either. So when you do talk, remember to plan to talk again, and soon. But set limits for how long you are going to talk. When the conversation is over, it's over, and should not be strung out over days and weeks.

And when you are planning the time to talk, plan the place, as well. As strange as this may sound, talking about sex shouldn't happen in the bedroom (or any other place where you have sex!). Find a neutral place and turn off the TV, the stereo, and the phone. Lock the front door. Make sure the dog has food and water and has been out for a walk. Interruptions can make a sensitive topic seem even more overwhelming and may break the flow of the discussion or may distract one or both of you from the task at hand.

Say the words.

Even though there are about 500 words used to describe the penis and testicles, most of them funny, it can be challenging to talk about this seriously with the person whom you love. It may be even stranger to talk about your partner's anatomy. Many men and women don't really know the "correct" names for the different parts of our anatomy. This in itself can cause embarrassment.

Some of us may only know the cute baby words we heard from our parents when we were young and then used with our own kids. But we feel embarrassed to use them when talking to our partners.

Try saying one of these words out loud: testicle. Say it again. Say it louder. It gets easier each time!

Name the problem.

You need to decide ahead of time what you want to talk about. And you need to be prepared to discuss it openly and honestly and constructively. This requires planning ahead, and it is a good idea to let your partner know what you want to talk about. Saying "Honey, we need to talk about our sex life" is too broad and may be confusing to the partner. What about your sex life? The frequency, the type of activity, your feelings about it? Be clear with your partner so that he or she can also do some thinking ahead of time. A better invitation may be "I would like to talk about the difficulties I've been having with erections lately."

Practice straight talk.

Talking about sex requires you to be clear in your words and expectations. Many of us think that our partner can or should be able to guess or intuit our needs and feelings. You may know each other very well, and you may be able to finish each others' sentences, and you may even think the same things at the same time, but if you want to solve a problem, then you need to be straightforward and clear about what you are thinking and feeling.

Tell your partner what you are feeling and why this is happening. The context is very important to avoid your partner thinking that the reason you are feeling this way is something that he or she has done. A vague statement such as "I have no desire for sex" may be interpreted as "He doesn't love or want me anymore." And what you mean is that since your surgery, you are very tired and just don't have the energy for sex right now.

Use the "I" word.

It is very important to talk about yourself and not put words in the mouth of your partner. That's not fair, and it won't help your conversation. If you need more direct stimulation since your surgery to get aroused, say something like, "I would love it if you would touch my penis with more pressure. Let me show you how I like it." That's much more constructive than saying "You don't know how to get me excited."

By talking in "I" statements you take ownership of your own feelings and don't put words in your partner's mouth or assume that you know what he or she is thinking or feeling. And from your partner's perspective, it doesn't feel like blame.

Balance the negative and the positive.

There are different ways of saying things, and how you say something can really influence how the message is received. "You make me crazy with your demands for sex" has a very different tone from "I don't want sex as often as you seem to." Sometimes when talking about sex, we have to say things that may seem hurtful or may appear to our partner as a criticism. Balancing the positive and the negative is a delicate negotiation but, if done carefully, can protect feelings and reduce the risk of causing hurt. If you find that your response to your partner's caress has changed, instead of stating the negative ("You don't know how to make me feel good"), you can be much more positive ("Let me show you where to touch me so that it feels really good").

Listen.

When your partner speaks, make the effort to listen, with both ears and your heart and mind. Don't think about the mess in the garage, what you have to do at work tomorrow, or that you've had the conversation before. Empty your mind of past memories and future plans, and truly listen.

Some couples find it useful to have a small item, such as a wooden spoon or other knickknack, for the person who's talking to hold. When one person is holding the item, it is that person's turn to talk, and he or she must not be interrupted until the item is given to the other person. This can help to focus the listener's attention because he or she cannot talk while the other person has the item.

One of the greatest gifts we can experience in our relationship is to be truly heard. So think about giving that gift to your partner by listening with your heart, mind, and soul.

Be flexible.

You may want something to be resolved in a certain way, but your partner may have different views. When talking about important subjects, we sometimes get defensive and stubborn, and then nothing gets solved. Give a little. When you are actively listening to your partner, let go of your own thoughts and opinions for a moment or two, and you may be surprised that your partner's position is not that far from yours. Many men are used to being listened to, but this is your relationship, and it takes two to make things better.

Get help.

Don't wait until you are faced with a crisis to get help. If every discussion ends up in a fight, you may need help. If every fight ends up with a week of silence, you need help. Marriage therapists and sex therapists or counselors are highly educated professionals who specialize in helping couples to understand what is affecting their relationship and, more importantly, helping them to find a better way of talking or reacting or loving.

Men often think that they have to solve every problem or crisis, and this extends into their relationships. Being part of a couple means that resolution of problems needs to be shared, so don't think you have to fix it—work on it together.

Communication is central to all our relationships. But we all need practice in getting it right.

CHAPTER 15

Where to Find Help

A number of resources are available that individuals and couples can use to help them through these trying times. This chapter provides information about where to get help and how to find and use resources that are useful.

Always be aware that books, magazines, and especially Web sites often contain personal anecdotes and experiences and may not be of the highest quality or scientifically valid.

Books

Men and Cancer

- Alterowitz, R., & Alterowitz, B. (2004). *Intimacy with impotence: The couple's guide to better sex after prostate disease.* Cambridge, MA: Da Capo Press.
- Fincannon, J.L., & Bruss, K.V. (2002). *Couples confronting cancer.* Atlanta, GA: American Cancer Society.
- Katz, A. (2007). *Breaking the silence on cancer and sexuality: A handbook for healthcare providers.* Pittsburgh, PA: Oncology Nursing Society.
- Laken, V., & Laken, K. (2002). *Making love again: Hope for couples facing loss of sexual intimacy.* Sandwich, MA: Ant Hill Press.
- Mulhall, J.P. (2008). *Saving your sex life: A guide for men with prostate cancer.* Munster, IN: Hilton Publishing.
- Perlman, G., & Drescher, J. (2005). *A gay man's guide to prostate cancer.* Binghamton, NY: Haworth Press.
- Schover, L. (1997). *Sexuality and fertility after cancer.* New York: John Wiley & Sons.

- Wainrib, B.R., Haber, S., & Maguire, J. (2000). *Men, women, and prostate cancer: A medical and psychological guide for women and the men they love* (2nd ed.). New York: New Harbinger Publications.

Male Sexuality

- Bader, M. (2008). *Male sexuality: Why women don't understand it—and men don't either.* Lanham, MD: Rowman & Littlefield Publishers.
- McCarthy, B.W., & Metz, M.E. (2008). *Men's sexual health: Fitness for satisfying sex.* New York: Routledge.
- Zilbergeld, B. (1999). *The new male sexuality* (Revised ed.). New York: Bantam.

Web Sites

- **Cancer Survivors Network**
  www.acscsn.org
  Vast amount of information related to surviving and thriving after cancer. Sponsored by the American Cancer Society.
- **Fertile Hope**
  www.fertilehope.org/index.cfm
  A national nonprofit organization dedicated to providing reproductive information, support, and hope to patients with cancer and survivors whose medical treatments present the risk of infertility
- **Institute of Medicine**
  www.iom.edu/CMS/3809/34252/47228.aspx
  Special section of the Institute of Medicine's Web site that addresses psychosocial health needs for people with cancer
- **National Sexuality Resource Center**
  www.nsrc.sfsu.edu
  Contains a wealth of information about sexuality for consumers and clinicians
- **OncoLink**
  www.oncolink.com/index.cfm
  Comprehensive cancer information for patients and their families

- **Out With Cancer**
  www.outwithcancer.com
  An online resource for gay, lesbian, bisexual, and transgendered people with cancer
- **Prostate Cancer Foundation**
  www.prostatecancerfoundation.org
  The foundation funds research into prostate cancer. The Web site highlights the latest information about prostate cancer.
- **The University of Texas M.D. Anderson Cancer Center**
  www.mdanderson.org/topics/sexuality
  Provides a range of articles about cancer and sexuality for men and women

Professional Counseling

- The American Association of Sexuality Educators, Counselors, and Therapists (www.aasect.org) has a list of qualified therapists and counselors across North America.